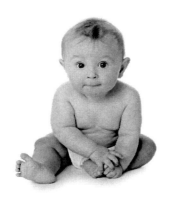

You Can Prevent Childhood Obesity

Practical Ideas from Pregnancy through Adolescence

Health: A Legacy for Our Children

Philip R. Nader, M.D.
Michelle Murphy Zive, M.S., R.D.

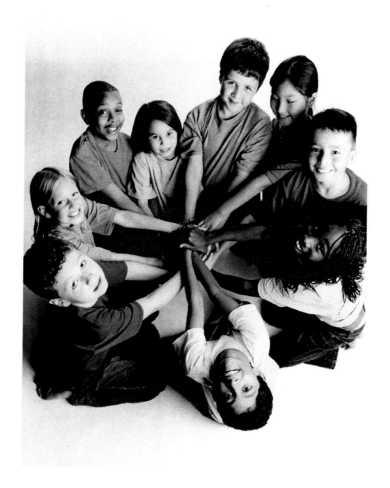

A **Legacy of Health** is the greatest gift we can give to our children.

Around the world, children from all cultural and ethnic backgrounds are currently in danger. No ethnic or cultural group is immune, all are affected. This book will help you understand some practical steps that we all can take to provide our children a **Legacy of Health**.

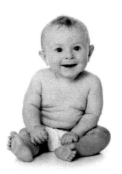

Busting America's Great Denial That Obesity Doesn't Affect Us

"Obesity, The Great Denial" was the title of an academic article published in the 1970s by a friend and mentor, Dr. Gilbert A. Forbes, at the University of Rochester, NY. Even then, this endocrinologist was pointing out how doctors and patients alike were in denial about the causes and effects of obesity.

This great denial is at the root of why, despite knowing better, many people hang on to **myths and misconceptions** that perpetuate the causes of overweight and obesity. These keep us from changing our own behavior and the behavior of others that could prevent the problem in the first place.

For example, because we don't really believe that obesity can affect us, we become complacent about advertising to our young, impressionable children; or we go along with cutting out physical activity and PE in schools because there is a greater need to emphasize academics.

We allow ourselves to buy into the **great denial** that "obesity" doesn't affect us, or our children.

"Obese" is a medical term – and one that we would certainly never use to refer to ourselves or our children! Instead we prefer to think we, or he, might just be carrying "a little extra weight." However, it takes only a little extra weight from pregnancy through adolescence to result in the epidemic of overweight that is predicted to affect 75% of adults and nearly 25% of kids by the year 2015.

There is another big economic reason why we buy into this **great denial: it is profitable to many parts of our society.** Obesity treatment specialists agree that prevention would be cheaper than treatment. Treatment is difficult, hard to sustain and costs a lot more than prevention. Sadly, people will spend more money and time on treatment than on prevention.

In this case, "an ounce" of prevention will not work; it will take at least a half a pound of prevention to equal a pound of cure! We all need to spend more time and money on preventing obesity.

Whether industries contribute to the causes of obesity, or deal with the consequences of obesity, all make billions each year. Most of us also have our eye on the "bottom line," and we know that making a profit supports the economy, but we must ask ourselves: at what cost?

We wrote this book so that you, as a parent, a health care provider, a business person, a politician, educator, or concerned citizen could understand the **myths and misconceptions** and act to **prevent this problem** rather than **treat** it. We provide simple **do's** and **don'ts** for each age and stage of child development from pregnancy through adolescence. Child development principles are key not only for parents, but also for marketing forces that use them to influence the consumption behaviors of youth.

There are many things that each and every one of us could do to change the environment back to being healthy. If we all did something, and did not do other things, then we could avoid monumental costs that are expected to easily top the costs to society we paid due to tobacco. More than that, we could avoid the real possibility that kids today will have a shorter life expectancy than their parents unless something is done.

Fighting the Great Denial (Second edition Preface)

The **Great Denial** about Obesity **continues today**. While most parents and many doctors see a "normal" infant or child, he or she has a good chance of really measuring as being overweight or obese. When we see an actually healthy weight child, we tend to think the child is "too skinny". **Most parents do not know that their overweight children are in fact overweight** – they think they are "normal", or will "outgrow their Baby Fat". That was the reason the first edition of this book was titled You Can Lose Your Baby Fat, but that title was confusing to many, thinking that the book was about post pregnancy weight loss for new Moms. This second edition has been updated with new research results and more tips and "clinical pearls", drawn from careful reviews of the first edition by practicing physicians and nurses. Gloria Sotelo M.D., has prepared the first cultural and language Spanish version "Usted Puede Prevenir Obesidad en los Niños, Ideas Prácticas del Embarazo a la Adolescencia."

Philip R. Nader, M.D.

Michelle M. Zive, M.S., R.D.

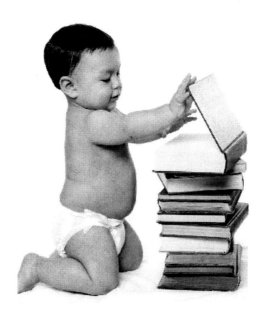

How To Read This Book

If you are a **Health Care Provider**, and already monitoring your patients weight, height and BMI, but you want concrete suggestions on how to counsel a family to increase activity and improve nutrition, we suggest you start with the appropriate chapters concerning the age of the child and the list of Do's and Don'ts for each stage found in Chapter 24.

Chapter 24 also includes "action plans" for modifying activity and nutrition behaviors. It includes forms which can be copied and developed jointly for each family.
(See www.youcanpreventchildhoodobesity.org) Chapter 24 has other handouts and tips for parents on portion size, shopping and monitoring BMI.

As a Health Care Provider you can advocate in your community to make the environment healthier for kids and families. You may also want to let your families know how to get a copy of the book for themselves by visiting www.youcanpreventchildhoodobesity.org.

If you are a **Parent or Prospective Parent,** we suggest you start with the section that closely matches where you are (e.g. pregnancy, toddler, school age, adolescence). Then go back and read through from the beginning. Pay attention to the many practical tips and nutrition, activity, and parenting skills that are sprinkled throughout.

If you are an **Early Childhood or School Educator**, you already appreciate that good health affects learning and vice versa. We suggest you read through the entire book, looking for practical ways you can improve the educational environment vis a vis nutrition and activity.

If you are in **Public Health, Government, Business, the Food Industry, Urban Planning, Transportation, Politics, Community Organizing, Media or other professions**, the authors applaud your interest in this topic. We urge you to read through the entire book to find ways in which your particular area of service can impact this major economic and health threat that affects all of us. You know your field. Armed with the knowledge you can gain in this book, you will be able to see opportunities to impact policies and practices that can help.

Table of Contents

Myths And Misconceptions

Preschool: Ages 2 to 4½

School: Ages 5 to 9

Tweens: Ages 9 to 12

Adolescence: Ages 12 to 17

Putting it All Together

1

MYTH:
You Can Lose Your Baby Fat

Ever heard this? "I'm not fat, just a little overweight."
"Look at the chubby baby, those little fat legs - isn't she cute?"
"Boy, he'll be a great football player - so big and tall at his age!"

These are all positive statements about being a little overweight. As a society, we have embraced a great denial about obesity and being overweight. This explains why most of us "might" be a "little" overweight. We can eat a little better; **when we have the time**, and exercise more; **when we have the time** and "obesity" need not concern us.

REALITY CHECK:

Being able to lose your baby fat might have been true thirty years ago, but not today! We can no longer cling to the denial that obesity will not affect our kids or us. Not with the way the environment has changed in the past thirty years.

Family photo albums are full of baby pictures showing the round-faced, cherubic, smiling baby. Turn the page and watch how the baby grows into a chubby toddler. Next, see the 10-year-old little leaguer, or the ballerina in her leotard thin and strong — no baby fat at all.

Then a picture of the same young woman in the one-piece bathing suit (we are talking thirty years ago), all curvy and attractive, or the fit young man poising with his tennis racket ready to slam a serve.

This possibility of "growing out of your baby fat" doesn't apply anymore because kids no longer grow up in the same kind of environment that kids used to.

MYTH BUSTER:

In a recent study that received a lot of press, entitled "Identifying Risk for Obesity in Early Childhood", 1000 children born in 1991, when the obesity epidemic was well under way, were measured for height and weight. Between the ages of 2 and 12 these children were measured seven times. The shocking news is: **The kids who were overweight even once during the preschool ages were five times more likely to be overweight at age 12 years than the kids who were never overweight from ages 2 to 4½ years.** These children, growing up during the obesity epidemic, did not lose their baby fat!

For the first time in history, children are faced with the possibility of having a shorter lifespan than their parents. Why is our society obsessed with protecting our children against the one-in-a-million chance of child abduction, and not against the one-in-three or four chances they have of developing obesity and being likely to die younger than their parents?

Are we saying that paying attention to the problem of children being abducted (mostly by relatives, by the way) is wrong? No, but we are saying that a comparable effort needs to be mounted to stop the way our children are raised today, which exposes them to far greater risks than being abducted.

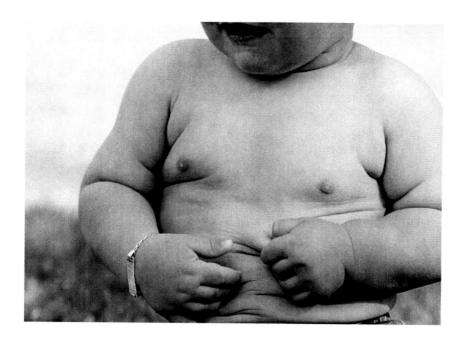

Some of the Stark Consequences of being Overweight in Childhood

- Children become isolated from their peers, learn that they cannot be active in sports, and develop low self esteem.

- Children develop physical ailments that were once reserved for overweight adults, such as sleeping, bone and joint problems, and high blood pressure, as well as liver disease (without ever taking a drop of alcohol).

- Today, there is an alarming increase in diabetes.

- This increase in diabetes is directly related to the increase in obesity.

- Overweight children are likely to become overweight adolescents and adults.

- All this adds up to a situation that, unless changed, will result in our children having a shorter life expectancy than we enjoy.

The proportion of overweight children has skyrocketed in the past thirty years! About 10% of kids were overweight in the 1970s, while today estimates are at least 30% overall, and even higher in some groups. Nearly half of adults are also overweight. While this epidemic may be leveling off, there are far too many kids and adults affected.

This rise in obesity has led experts to predict costs to society in medical complications and lost work rivaling, if not exceeding, the costs to society that tobacco was responsible for.

Even if your children are already raised, or you or your family are not directly affected by this problem, you pay taxes and health insurance, so you have a stake in doing something about the problem.

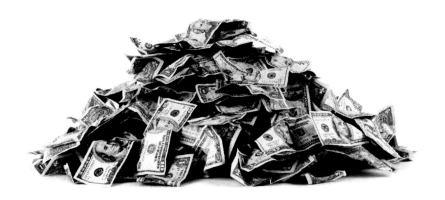

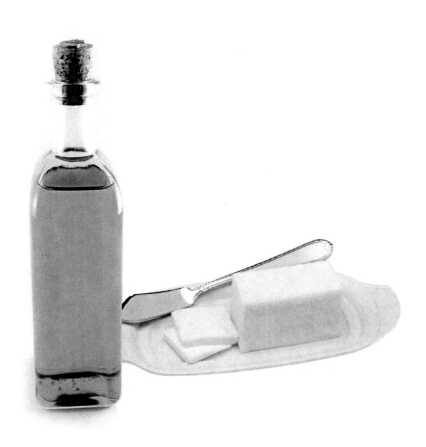

2

MISCONCEPTION:
All Fat is Bad:
The Skinny on Fat

Ever heard this? "Just read the label: reduced fat!"
"Lose weight by eating more fat."

No wonder people are confused!

The great denial about being overweight carries over into the presumed causes of being fat in the first place. Our society has also demonized fat and its various forms as all being bad. This game has led to fad diets that include heavy amounts of fat, all grapefruit, and other impossible and unhealthy-to-sustain nutritional adventures.

REALITY CHECK:

Fat performs an important role in our bodies. It stores energy for us, provides protection and insulation, and cushions organs and bones from injury. Fat is actually an organ itself, composed of adipose tissue or fat cells.

New fat cells are developed at four times during the life cycle:

- **The last three months of gestation in the womb and the early months of infancy**
- **Early childhood ages 4-6 years**
- **Adolescence**
- **Pregnancy for child bearing women**

These are the only times that new fat cells increase in number. At all other times, adipose tissue gets larger by adding fat to the inside of already existing fat cells. The fat cells get larger when the body gets more calories in than it expends in energy to move around, maintain the body and grow. Fat cells chemically demand to be kept full. That is why adult weight loss can be difficult.

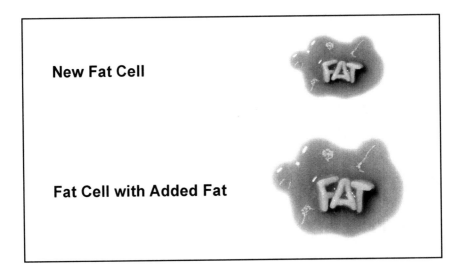

New Fat Cell

Fat Cell with Added Fat

That is also why fat babies become overweight children who become overweight teens and adults. There is a constant excess of energy in verses energy out. This is called an imbalance in the energy equation.

The Gene-Environment Interaction

How and Why does Fat Accumulate in Fat Cells? It is because of the interaction between genes and the environment. An amazing and pretty recent example can be found in the Aboriginal people of Australia. Up until the beginning of the twentieth century, Aboriginals were isolated from advancing civilization, and kept an extremely thin body type inherited from many generations of low-fat, low-protein intake. In the 1970s, a health study was done among the Aboriginal population in Australia: there was no diabetes and people lived to an old age. Today, an Aboriginal person who looks like an average sized non-native person is actually many times more "obese" than their parents or grandparents were, even several decades ago. Diabetes is now rampant, and the life expectancy is around 40 to 50 years, with end-stage renal disease from diabetes the major culprit. Civilization moves much faster than evolution and adaptation.

Today we are faced with a similar paradox: our bodies are ready to save fat for a rainy day, while we not only have more than enough to eat, we are also much less active than our ancestors — or even our grandparents — were.

Label Definitions

When you read labels you need to understand what the rules are for putting certain claims on foods. The government says what various claims must mean:

Claims for Calories

Calorie free:	Less than 5 calories per serving
Low calorie:	40 calories or less per serving

Claims for Fat

Fat free:	Less than 0.5 gram of fat or saturated fat per serving
Saturated fat free:	Less than 0.5 gram of saturated fat per serving
Low fat:	3 grams or less of total fat
Low saturated fat:	1 gram or less of saturated fat
Reduced fat or less fat	At least 25% less fat than the original version

Claims for Sugar

Sugar free:	Less than 0.5 gram of sugar per serving
Reduced sugar:	At least 25% less sugar per serving than the original version

Claims for Fiber

High fiber:	5 grams or more of fiber per serving
Good source of fiber:	2.5 to 4.9 grams of fiber per serving

Science has found it difficult to pin the blame on a single culprit for the imbalance (more calories in than out) in the energy equation. Take fast foods, for example. While it is true that people who consume fast foods get more calories and less nutritional value than those who do not, one study found that both overweight and lean teenagers ate similar amounts of fast food, yet the lean teenagers compensated with more activity and healthier other foods, compared to the overweight ones.

MYTH BUSTER:

People who live in neighborhoods with a blend of shops and businesses within an easy walk have a 35% lower risk of obesity. This is the antithesis of suburban sprawl with shops and businesses that are driving distance away. People who achieve the well-advertised ideal of living in the idyllic suburban setting with no sidewalks, and nothing but garages facing the street, will of necessity get in their car to do just about anything, even drive to their mail box. These folks automatically increase their risk of obesity just by where they live!

Why has the energy equation become out of kilter?

Most likely the problem is that the environment has changed dramatically over the past several decades, especially with regard to how and what we eat, and the opportunities we have to be active. Just talk with your parents or grandparents to discover the many ways society has changed our habits.

What Happened? A lot!

- TV trays make it easier for us to sit in front of the TV and eat.
- TV dinners are an easy replacement for home-cooked meals and make it easier to sit in front of the TV and eat.
- The number of television sets per household, and particularly in bedrooms, has increased.
- Corn syrup was introduced as a universal sweetener.
- Soft drinks and juice drinks have increased in availability and been heavily marketed.
- High calorie, high fat snacks and fast food restaurants became more available, and not surprisingly, intake has increased.
- Fast food outlets have been marketed to children by enticing them with toys and games.
- Fewer meals are eaten at home.
- Super-sized meals and big portion sizes have become common.
- Now 80% of kids ride to school rather than 80% walking to school.
- There are fewer parks and available safe places for kids to play.
- There is much greater reliance upon car travel, even for short distances.
- The layout of housing developments, in isolated communities, requires cars.

- There have been changes in school and day care environments, including offering of sodas and unhealthy snacks.
- There have been huge increases in advertising supporting inactivity (buy video games) and unhealthy eating (buy sugary cereals).
- School physical education has been reduced: only 5% of kids have daily PE.
- Recess in schools has been reduced or eliminated.
- There is more childcare, and earlier childcare.
- There has been a general increase in the amount of TV watched and other screen time.
- There are more employed and out-of-home parents.

MYTH BUSTER:

Fact: Half of all ad time on children's shows is taken up with food ads. More facts: 34% of ads focus on candy and snacks, 28% on cereal, and 10% on fast food. Only 4% highlight dairy products (milk), 1% promote fruit juices, and zero are for fruits and vegetables. The power of advertising over young children's choices is amazing. In one study, young kids preferred a rock with a recognizable cartoon character on it to a delicious snack without it. No wonder millions of dollars are spent on advertising to children. Ask any parent who takes a young child to the supermarket if advertising works!

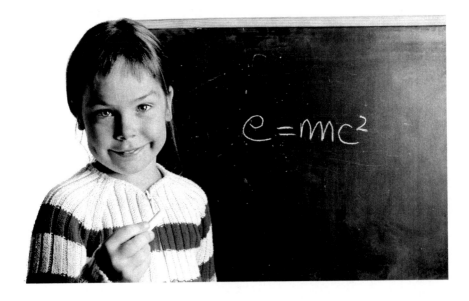

3

MISCONCEPTION:
Overweight is Too Complex to Understand and Prevent

Ever heard this? "I heard about this great new diet!"
"Nobody is sure what causes overweight; it's all too complex."
"We know that immunizations work, we don't know if overweight can be prevented." (from a doctor)

Our search for a quick fix, the magic pill, six-minute abs, and a painless way to become slim and attractive leads our society to spend millions of dollars every year on trying to lose weight. If only someone had told us that preventing overweight in the first place would keep us on a path that would not require a search for the magic "cure."

REALITY CHECK:

Understanding why people get overweight is not rocket science! The basic reason why people put on extra weight is found in the basic energy equation. That is, the energy taken in equals the energy expenditure required for activity, maintaining and growing the body. If more energy is taken in than is expended, the body gains weight.

The table below shows the actual number of extra pounds it takes to medically classify a child as overweight or obese, according to guidelines used by doctors.

You will be surprised how very little extra weight for a girl of average height at younger ages can put her at risk for later overweight: (The numbers are similar for boys.)

Age	Normal weight in pounds	Extra pounds to be overweight	Extra pounds to be obese
3	32	+4 = 36	+6 = 38
7	55	+3 = 58	+ 10 = 65
12	104	+15 = 119	+ 34 = 138

You can see that only a few extra pounds puts you at risk of obesity when you are younger. That is the bad news, but the good news is that it should be easier then to stop the gradual putting on of extra weight by limiting intake of sweets and fats and increasing the amount of play and activity, rather than waiting until later, when it will be much more difficult for the child to "grow into" the extra weight.

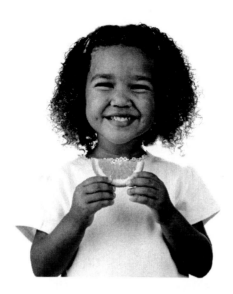

How can you tell if your child is on the way to becoming overweight?

You used to be able to just look at them, but that is no longer the case. This is true for both lay people and doctors!

Up to age two, you can look at the routine growth charts your doctor uses. You will be able to see on the chart where your child is for both height and weight, in comparison to other babies. If your baby is, say, at the 50th percentile for height, but at the 90th percentile for weight, that means that he is gaining more weight than he needs compared to his height.

This does not mean you should put him on a "diet." However, it does warrant a review of what you are feeding your child, how much and how often. **Babies who gain weight quickly in the first year of life tend to hang on to that extra weight.**

BMI — Body Mass Index

After the age of two, BMI can be used to track the amount of excess weight for a given height and gender, over time. To get your child's BMI number from their age, gender and current weight and height, visit the Centers for Disease Control and Prevention website at: http://cdc.gov/nccdphp/dnpa/bmi/. You can calculate it yourself using the formula: weight (kg)/ [height (m)]^2.

By looking at the BMI charts for girls and boys on pages 20 and 21, you can tell if a child is "underweight" (less than the 5th percentile), "normal" (between the 5th and 85th percentile), "overweight" (85th to less than the 95th percentile), or "obese" (95th percentile or over).

By marking your child's BMI on the BMI charts in this book every year (maybe on their birthday or on New Year's Day), you can see how well you are doing at monitoring their energy balance, and keeping them in the normal range.

If your child does creep into the overweight category, it is a good idea to try to improve the energy balance while they are still young, as the tendency is to keep weight on or add, rather than to lose it.

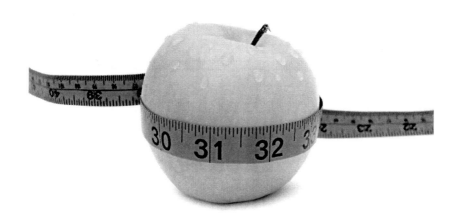

Body Mass Index

Under Weight	Less than 5th percentile
Normal Weight	Between 5th and 85th percentile
Over Weight	Between 85th and 95th percentile
Obese	95th percentile and over

CDC Growth Charts: United States

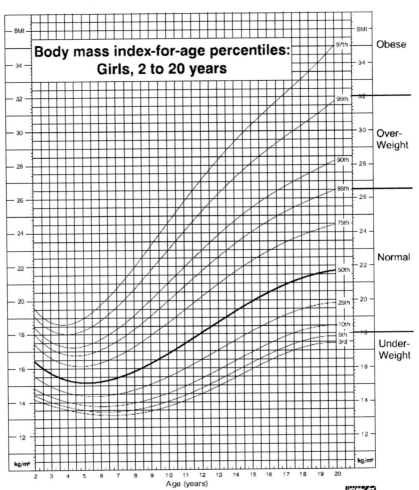

Body mass index-for-age percentiles:
Girls, 2 to 20 years

Obese

Over-Weight

Normal

Under-Weight

97th
95th
90th
85th
75th
50th
25th
10th
5th
3rd

BMI

34

32

30

28

26

24

22

20

18

16

14

12

kg/m²

Age (years)

Published May 30, 2000.
SOURCE: Developed by the National Center for Health Statistics in collaboration with
the National Center for Chronic Disease Prevention and Health Promotion (2000).

SAFER · HEALTHIER · PEOPLE™

CDC Growth Charts: United States

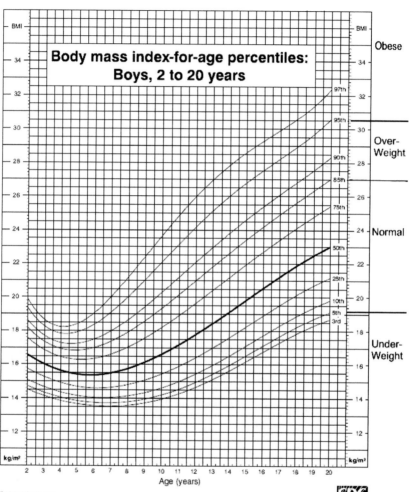

Body mass index-for-age percentiles: Boys, 2 to 20 years

Published May 30, 2000.
SOURCE: Developed by the National Center for Health Statistics in collaboration with
the National Center for Chronic Disease Prevention and Health Promotion (2000).

SAFER · HEALTHIER · PEOPLE™

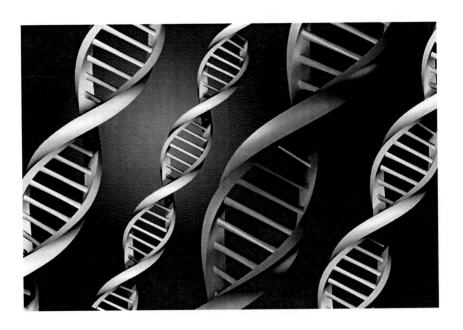

4

MYTH:
Obesity Is All Due To Genetics

Ever heard this? "You can't blame the environment. I know for a fact that obese people are just lazy and from broken homes."

"Being overweight runs in our family; there's nothing to be done."

"It's a problem with my metabolism."

"I can gain weight on water!"

REALITY CHECK:

Genetics and Metabolism

Less than 5% of overweight and obese children have a diagnosable "metabolic" or "glandular" cause for being overweight. About 25–40% of the tendency to become overweight is "heritable" (that means due to the genes). If both your parents are obese, you have a greater chance of becoming obese, but 60–75% of the cause of your own overweight comes back to imbalance in the energy equation

— i.e. taking in more calories than you burn. It's also true that identical twins raised separately have remarkably similar weight status, but even those identical twins raised apart still have remarkably similar exposures to advertising, fast foods, empty calories and lack of physical activity.

Family History Scan

This exercise will help you determine the possible genetic risks that you and your partner might face. Look at some family photo albums!

Find out about genetic risks in your family by talking with parents and grandparents, and aunts and uncles. The presence or absence of obesity, or being overweight can increase the manifestation of certain disease risks such as diabetes, heart attacks, strokes, and high blood pressure. In general, the younger individuals are when they have these medical conditions (especially before age fifty), the more serious the threat. The family history scan applies to both prospective parents, but only to your biological relatives.

A last word on the Gene-Environment Interaction: Since genes do play a role in susceptibility to being overweight, it is possible that as the overweight youth of today become parents themselves, genetics will become more important, unless something is done to address the current energy imbalance. **Remember, genetics did not change in the past thirty years, but the environment sure did!**

REALITY CHECK:

Broken Homes and Laziness

As a pediatrician and a nutritionist we have seen an unfortunately large number of physically and sexually abused children who develop life-long consequences of poor self-image, and self-destructive behaviors including eating too much or not enough. However, people who are overweight are not all victims of disadvantage, poverty, or broken homes.

People who are overweight also are not intrinsically lazy, or unmotivated. They have not necessarily suffered from a traumatic childhood. When nearly half of adults and a third of kids are overweight or obese, there is no way you can blame the problem on a single thing: not genes, not parenting, not the schools. Instead it's an accumulation of all of these factors that makes it easier now, especially among susceptible individuals, to be overweight than to be fit and healthy.

That isn't to say that parenting has no role in determining the eventual weight status of kids. Family dynamics often affect eating and activity habits. What happens in life to children as they grow up sets up complicated relationships that influence their activity and eating habits. These habits in turn influence whether a child is underweight, normal weight, overweight or obese.

Think Back

Were you a fussy eater? Did your parents yell at you to eat more? Did you have scary feelings in your stomach when forced to eat? What effect has that had on your own dietary habits today? Given those feelings, if you can recall them, how are you likely to handle a fussy eater who is your own child?

The intended or unintended messages that children get can have a big impact on them. Did you get a clear message that to be a proper young lady you should sit quietly, pursue intellectual and artistic activities, and certainly not sweat? Do you think that had a lasting effect on your enthusiasm for exercise and activity? If you, as a young boy, were somewhat afraid of the rough and tumble ways of some of your peers, did that make it less likely that you tried and mastered different sports?

There is very little research on parenting and obesity. But what is out there suggests that over-controlling parenting and lack of sensitivity to the child may be factors leading to being overweight or obese. This means that you need to be able to be **responsive to the type of child you get.** They are all different, as anyone knows who has had more than one child in a family! Recognizing these individual differences will allow you to read the child's cues and communicate. This will help shape their emerging nutrition and activity habits.

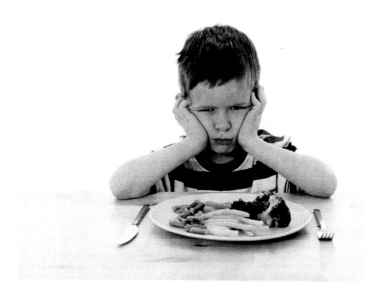

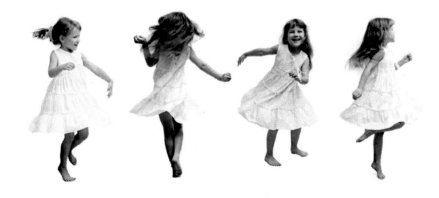

5

MYTH:
A Quiet Child is a Good Child

Ever heard or said this? "Slow down!"

"Be careful!"

"Sit down!"

"Go watch some TV — you're driving me crazy!"

REALITY CHECK:

Most kids are naturally active.

They run, climb, jump, dance … until you think you might go crazy. This activity burns energy, and is nature's way of shifting the energy balance in the kid's favor — more energy is burned than put into their mouths.

This kind of activity builds strength, increases agility and speed of reflexes, and builds self-confidence in the body and what it can do. Kids spend more combined time in front of the

TV or playing computer or console games than at school. This means that the average kid has three to five or more hours per day of screen time during the week, and as much on the weekends, thus totaling more hours than schooling itself! If most of the school and leisure time is sedentary, what happens to the energy equation? You guessed it.

> **MYTH BUSTER:**
> Study after study show that the more time preschoolers spend outdoors, the higher their activity levels. Other factors shown in studies to increase activity levels include prompts from peers and adults to be active.

We do our kids a huge disservice by discouraging activity and dampening their enthusiasm for channeling their energy. Some children are naturally coordinated, or have a genetic background that will make them star athletes.

However, some of us are not the most coordinated people. If your child is less coordinated, or less active, than other children, then you need to guide them to activities they like — and not necessarily the ones you think they should be doing.

There are too many examples of parents hoping their children will be a star football player or tennis player, when the child lacks the ability and more importantly the passion to be what the parents want.

Don't over think the physical activity stuff. Kids will be kids. Let them be just that and run around burning all those calories. Play sets the stage for an active life. Get the kids off to an early start with play and being active.

Tim Haft, a trainer, illustrates this point: "When Suzy came to me she was 35, five feet tall, and weighed 210 pounds. She'd been sedentary most of her life. Her parents and other family members never encouraged her to play, exercise, or participate in sports, and I suspect she had little opportunity to be active at school, like in PE classes. She became comfortable being stationary. This is the killer. Once you're comfortable not moving, and once you gain a significant amount of weight, the odds are really stacked against you in terms of reversing the trend." Since Suzy has been involved in a regular exercise program, she's lost 60 pounds.

Activity should be fun! If you, as the parent, see exercise and activity as necessary, but is something you dread, it is unlikely that it will be incorporated into your lifestyle. And if you feel this way, certainly your children will view activity in the same way.

Since less than half of adults exercise on a regular basis, some changes have to be made to make the next generation more likely to be active on a daily basis compared to their parents.

What are some simple things the family can do to encourage activity?

- Mark on the calendar when you will take a walk together as a family. Or you walk and let the kids ride their tricycles or bicycles.

- Have family outings at the park, beach or lake. Play games like tag, volleyball or soccer.

- On the weekends, turn off the TV and go out and play with your children. When was the last time, you played on a jungle gym? See who can slide down the slide the fastest. Try to keep moving for a least a half hour.

- Role model. Your kids will learn more about being active by seeing you taking the time to go for a run or walk, or doing yoga. Another myth we'd like to bust is the old adage, "Do as I say, not as I do." This is never a good parenting strategy, especially when the health of your child is at stake.

- Encourage them to play outside whenever they can. Not safe? Or are your children too young to go out on their own? Then make it a priority to take the time and go outside with them to supervise.

If you yourself are an adult who has not learned to enjoy activity, and are not likely to change your own habits, you do not have to leave that legacy to your children! Look for other adults who can encourage, model and coach your children to be active and enjoy physical activity — this could be a local YMCA, Parks and Recreation Department, or school PE teacher. There are still things you can do to be more active, like taking the stairs instead of the elevator, buying a cheap pedometer and walking at least 10,000 steps a day, parking far away from the mall or grocery store, or doing household chores that burn energy... wash the car, rake leaves, or do the laundry. Even better, get your children involved; this will increase the fun factor. They'll benefit from being more physical and they'll learn about sharing in the responsibility of helping around the house.

The Vicious Cycle of Inactivity and Obesity

As we pack on the pounds, we are less likely to be active. Try a little experiment: fill a backpack with lots of heavy books. Try to get the weight up to 40 pounds or more. Now put it on and go about your daily activities. Doesn't feel too good, does it? Now imagine wearing the backpack all day every day and you don't like being active in the first place. You'd find it boring. Do you think you'd be likely to get out there and start exercising now? This is the daily reality for 50% of Americans. And once we're adults, it's really tough to escape this vicious cycle.

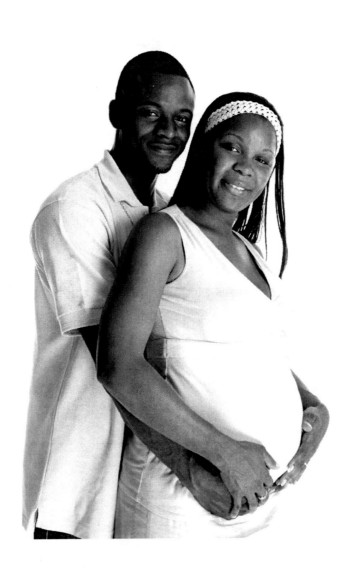

6

MYTH:
You're Pregnant...
You Can Eat For Two!

Ever heard this? "I just want a dish of ice cream and some
                 pickles!"
                 "Oh, another brownie won't matter."
                 "I'm so exhausted, I just want to sit here!"
                 "I can't see my shoes, anyway!"

REALITY CHECK:

Now you are pregnant, you can eat for two!

Better not! Excess weight gain during pregnancy has been
associated in research studies with extra weight later in
childhood through adulthood. Also, since pregnancy is
associated with a time of increasing numbers of fat cells, it
may be harder to lose weight put on during pregnancy.

In the old days, the really old days (we're talking thousands of years ago), additional fat cells were laid down during pregnancy as a safeguard against starvation for both the mother and the growing baby.

Nowadays, instead of waiting for hubby to kill the saber tooth tiger and drag it home so his pregnant partner can get some protein for her developing baby, we just have to stop off at the local supermarket. Our hunting and gathering society today means driving to the supermarket and hunting for what we desire or think we desire as a result of advertising!

Michelle Zive says: "Take it from a mom who gained 65, 45 and 70 pounds with each of my pregnancies and had gestational diabetes with my first: my children are now more at risk for being overweight and having diabetes later in life. On top of that, it took me forever to lose the weight. In fact, here I am three years after the birth of Jack and I'm still trying to get back to my pre-pregnancy weight."

Weight gain occurs during pregnancy, but the amount and timing of weight gain can be monitored and altered with adherence to recommendations received from your OB-GYN, family physician, or nurse.

The amount of recommended weight gain depends upon your initial body mass index or BMI. For the average weight woman (BMI 19.8–26.0), about one pound per week during the second and third trimesters — or a total of about 25–35 pounds — is suggested. If carrying twins, a slightly larger weight gain is expected. **These guidelines have been revised for the first time in several decades. Be sure to check with your doctor for the latest recommendations regarding ideal weight during pregnancy.**

Excessive overweight during pregnancy has serious consequences for both the mother and the baby. Again, best practice suggests early and regular pre-natal care.

On the flipside is a potential side-effect of society's preoccupation with thinness (there's a lot of irony there): not enough weight gain during pregnancy may cause fetal under nutrition and low birth-weight infants. This is a potentially preventable cause of low birth weight.

Again, nature tells us that the balance is what is important: needs vs. intake. Pregnancy increases the needs, so a normal pregnancy and response will result in normal weight gain. It is the excesses on either end — not enough weight gain or too much — that leads to an unhealthy weight for the baby.

Healthy eating for two: What pregnant women need to eat, not just want to eat.

As mentioned, pregnancy doesn't mean eating twice as much food. The recommendation is that pregnant women consume only **300 more calories a day.** (Note: You may not need this many calories during the first three months of your pregnancy.) Getting an additional 300 calories per day is very easy to do. A medium bagel (3½ inches diameter) is almost 300 calories; a carton of yogurt is 120.

Keep in mind that the "extra" calories you choose should come from nutrient dense foods, that is, foods that contain loads of fiber, vitamins and minerals.

How should your diet change during your pregnancy? The American Dietetic Association recommends that pregnant women consume approximately 2500–2700 calories per day. The range depends on your age, your starting weight and your physical activity level. Most pregnant women do well on a 2500-calorie diet.

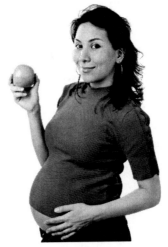

What does a 2500-calorie diet look like? Below are the kinds of foods and numbers of servings per day you'll need.

- 9 servings of breads and cereals. Choose whole grains to increase your fiber intake. Servings include 1 slice of bread, ¾ cup of whole-grain cereal, ½ cup of rice, cooked cereal or pasta.

- 7 servings of fruits and vegetables. The more "color" a fruit or a vegetable has, the more nutrients it has. (Think of the light green color of iceberg lettuce compared to the deep green of spinach.) Servings include: 1/2 cup of cooked broccoli, 2 small oranges, ½ cup of cut-up papaya.

- 3 servings of dairy. Choose non-fat or low-fat dairy products, such as skim milk or 1% yogurt. Servings include: 1 cup of milk, 8 ounces of yogurt, 1 ounce of natural cheese such as cheddar.

- 3 servings of protein. Choose low-fat sources of protein such as skinless chicken breast, lean or extra lean beef, and dried beans (which are high in fiber, too). Servings include: 1 egg, or a piece of meat the size of deck of cards.

Example of a Day's Menu

Breakfast	Snack	Lunch	Snack	Dinner
2 slices of whole-wheat toast	1½ ounces of low-fat mozzarella cheese	1 turkey sandwich with 3 ounces of turkey, 1 ounce slice of cheddar cheese, 2 whole-grain pieces of bread, green leafy lettuce and sliced tomatoes	1 cup of skim milk	3 ounces of salmon
2 table-spoons peanut butter	4 whole-grain crackers		½ bagel with low-fat cream cheese	½ cup of brown rice
½ mango				½ cup of steamed broccoli
½ cup of orange juice		2 cups of salad with low-fat dressing or olive oil and balsamic vinegar		1 whole-wheat roll

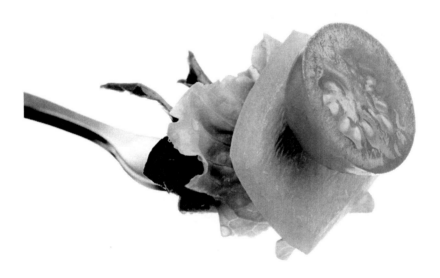

Tips for Healthy Eating During Pregnancy

- Have healthy food available in the home. This is the kind of thing that should continue after your baby is born. Have cut-up fruit in the refrigerator. Wash and drain spinach leaves for an easy-to-make salad. Have almonds and whole-grain bread in your cupboard. You're more likely to eat better, and later your children will too, if your home is set up to make eating healthy easy.

- Drink at least 32 ounces of water.

- Fill up on fiber by eating whole-grain breads and cereals, as well as dried beans, legumes and nuts.

- Eat every 3 to 4 hours. This will maintain your blood sugar level, you'll have more energy throughout the day, and you'll be less likely to binge.

Eat sweets and fats every once in a while. Treat yourself to low-fat frozen yogurt instead of ice cream. Instead of eating the entire candy bar, eat half of it. Choose baked chips instead of regular chips. You've seen what happens when you try to deny yourself that candy bar — you end up eating three instead of the one you wanted in the first place.

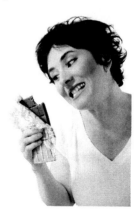

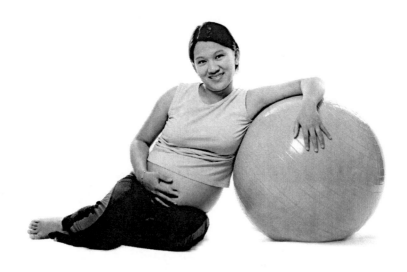

7

MISCONCEPTION:
Be Careful About Exercise and Sex During Pregnancy

Ever heard this? "Don't run or work out if you are pregnant."

"Oh honey, not tonight, I'm too tired."

"Don't you find me attractive now that I'm pregnant?"

REALITY CHECK:

The importance of early and regular pre-natal care cannot be overemphasized. In addition to health care, it is a good idea to look at your lifestyle and other habits. Routine daily exercise, adequate sleep, stress avoidance and parenting education are all helpful when considering pregnancy. If you smoke, you will never find a more important time or reason to quit.

Seek out support from family and friends to avoid drugs and alcohol if you think you are pregnant, or are planning pregnancy. The investment you put into your own health and well-being will pay dividends not only to you but also to your child.

Another word on physical activity: walking during and after pregnancy is a great way to limit the effects of eating "for two," and will also counter the tendency to cut down on your normal active lifestyle during and after pregnancy.

MYTH BUSTER:

Sexual activity is a normal form of physical exertion that most experts agree can be continued throughout pregnancy, especially if your pregnancy is normal and "low risk." Your OB or nurse can advise you further. But just because you can have sex doesn't necessarily mean you want it. Expect either an increase or decrease in desire — both are normal. The important thing is to keep open communication with your partner on the topic.

In addition to taking good care of yourself during pregnancy, this is a period when you have some time to consider what things you want to emphasize in order for your children to grow up as healthy as they can. This can include decisions about immunizations and child-rearing. Breast feeding classes should be started during pregnancy.

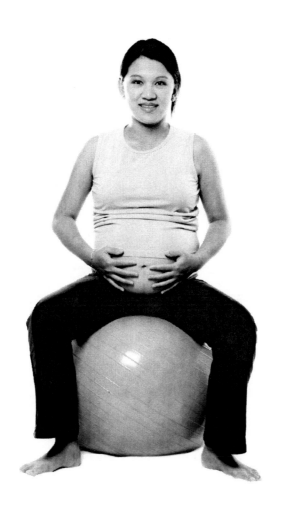

See Chapter 24 for a Summary of Do's and Don'ts for Pregnancy.

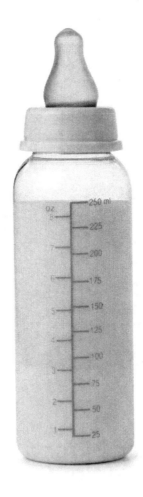

8

MYTH:
There's No Difference Between Breast and Bottle

Ever heard this? "I would breastfeed, but I want to go back to work."

"I don't know, breastfeeding seems so … primitive!"

"My husband wants to share in feeding the baby."

"Breastfed babies look so skinny!"

REALITY CHECK:

Track record: 600 million years of breastfeeding verses 60 years of bottle/formula feeding. Bottle feeding was a lifesaver in the 1800s for orphans and abandoned infants who would have died because there was no mother or wet-nurse to breastfeed them.

This may be the first time you become aware that you might be bombarded by people around you to not do the right thing by your child. Formula companies spend millions of dollars in advertising (such as hospital formula giveaways) to try to get you to feed your child formula. Many hospital staff are not trained to provide adequate support for breastfeeding, which does not help mothers who are unaware of the nutritional and other benefits of breastfeeding. Some men and fathers have attitudes against breastfeeding. All these forces counter traditional cultural beliefs that support breastfeeding.

MYTH BUSTER:

There are less than forty hospitals in the United States that are certified baby-friendly; that have programs to promote breastfeeding and a track record of doing so. This means that parents who want to breastfeed need to be extra-active in getting support.

MYTH BUSTER:

If one were to ask which formula is closest to mother's breast milk, the correct answer is none are similar to human milk – they all have casein, whey, calcium and phosphorus and even a few have corn syrup.

Exclusive breastfeeding is by far the best way to meet the nutritional needs of the growing baby — for as long as is practical. **Six months is recommended.**

However, even a short duration — 3 weeks to 3 months — of only breastfeeding has a biologic value by providing proteins that fight infection. Some research suggests that breastfeeding protects against obesity later in life. Not all studies agree, since it is really difficult to accurately determine the real length of exclusive breastfeeding.

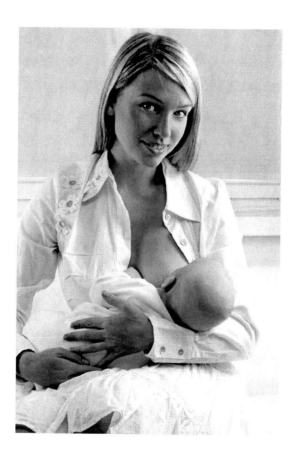

Tips to Improve Your Chances of Breastfeeding Successfully

- Find a support mom who has successfully breastfed.

- Start breastfeeding within the first hour after birth. The baby needs the colostrum which is the first fluid from the breast.

- Drink plenty of water and eat a well-balanced diet.

- Know that your milk will "come in" in 3-4 days. baby is born with a safety water and nutrition supply until then.

- Relax and enjoy the experience. That means finding a quiet place with a pillow to prop up your arms.

- If you're having a problem, call your support person.

- Try different positions to breastfeed that you and your baby like.

- Get a good "latch" by having baby have as much of your areola in her mouth as possible.

- Switch the breast that you initiate breastfeeding each time.

- Within 48–72 hours of initiating breastfeeding, seek evaluation of your breastfeeding technique by a trained professional or your support person.

- Feed your baby when he or she shows signs of hunger. This is the first example of you as a parent offering the "food" and your child letting you know when to feed. In the first few months this is usually every 2-3 hours.

- Nurse until your baby is satisfied: This usually means they've turned away from the breast or released their lips from the nipple. Ten or fifteen minutes on each side is usually sufficient. Some babies are more efficient than others.

- Avoid a hard rubber nipple when establishing breast feeding. A soft pacifier can be used if baby wants to suck in between feeds.

- Burp your baby at natural breaks, switching breasts during breastfeeding.

- Breastfeed your child exclusively for at least the first six months. Don't supplement with formula, water, vitamin or glucose water.

Start breast-feeding at first every 2-3 hours to stimulate milk production. Then, every 3-4 hours, for 10 minutes or so (depending on your baby) on each breast. This is adequate intake for the first six months of life.

Learn to read cues from your baby as to when the baby has had enough! Breastfed babies can be "overfed" by adding a bottle after the baby finishes the breast.

If you are using only bottle feeding, formula should not exceed 32 ounces a day. Picture this: a baby, with a bottle in the mouth, turning to the side, wrinkling up her face, "thinking": "Geez, Mom. Can't you tell when I'm full?"

Disadvantages of Bottle Feeding

- Cost

- Greater risks due to infections and possibly other chronic diseases

- Greater chance of becoming allergic to cow's milk

- Less ability to know when the baby has had "enough" milk

- It's tempting to want the baby to "finish the bottle", so there's more danger of overfeeding

The "formula" for successful infant feeding is not that difficult — keep on the track of normal weight gain, and allow the baby to call the shots on when to feed. Learn to read the way that babies signal that they have had enough for that feeding by turning away or clamping the mouth shut.

Returning to Work

Every attempt should be made to reach the goal of exclusive breastfeeding for the first six months. You probably can't take your baby to work with you, but that need not mean having to switch to formula.

Know your rights! Many states now require work sites to provide facilities where lactating working mothers can pump breast milk and store it safely to feed to their breastfeeding infants. It need not be an overly elaborate facility: a screened off corner that is quiet, private and clean, with a comfortable chair, is all that is required. Mothers can bring the bottles and a cooled container for storage. It is better for your baby to be fed breast milk in a bottle rather than formula when you are not present. If your employer is resistant, see if other fellow employees would support your request for adequate facilities to pump your breasts.

If Breast Feeding is Not Possible

Many babies have grown up physically and emotionally healthy and never breastfed. Therefore, if for some reason, it is not possible to breastfeed your infant, do not despair that you will place your baby in irreparable harm! Because formula from a bottle is much easier for the baby to suck and get full on, a feeding every 3 to 4 hours, even for the newborn, will last. A good number to remember as a maximum is 32 ounces per 24 hours. If the baby seems to want more, avoid overfeeding formula and substitute a bottle of water.

Try to be aware of the cues that baby is full, especially if he turns away. Avoid trying to "empty" the bottle every time if the baby doesn't want it. Watch the growth charts to observe the relationship between weight gain and length gain.

As the infant gets older and solid foods are introduced, and when he can hold a cup, formula can be switched to milk. Do not use a bottle of milk or juice to pacify during the day or at night or put a baby to bed with the bottle.

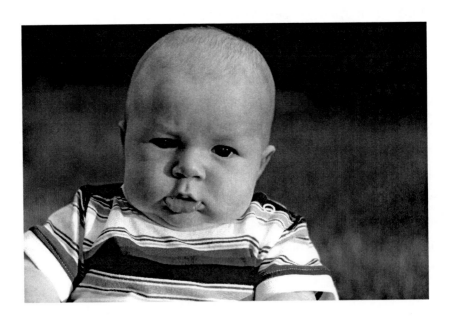

9

MYTH:
A Chubby Baby
Means A Healthy Baby
And A Good Mom

Ever heard this? "What a cute baby (cherubic, round-
faced, pudgy thighs)!"
"Gonna be a football player!"
"You must be so proud."

REALITY CHECK:

Everybody loves the plump, smiling baby — so cuddly! You
feel like a successful mom when your baby attracts this
positive attention. Having a chubby baby used to mean in
some cultures that the family was affluent enough to give
more than adequate food to their offspring!

However, chubby now does not necessarily mean healthy
later. The baby's weight status can easily be checked on

growth charts in your doctor's office. Watch to be sure that the baby's weight is not increasing faster than the distance between the percentile lines on the chart. For a normal infant, a weight gain averaging over an ounce a day may lead to an overweight situation. Several decades ago we used to teach young doctors that by 5 or 6 months babies would double their birth weight. Now this is likely to happen as early as 3–4 months. This is most likely due to patterns of overfeeding. Remember, more calories in than is needed for growth means more fat stored on your baby. That takes quite a lot of extra calories, because growth needs are never greater than in infancy.

> Studies have shown that 12-month-old infants who were above the 95th percentile for weight were more likely to become overweight adolescents and adults.

Feeding the baby is a way that mothers can prove that they are adequate. Therefore, how satisfied the baby seems and the visual appearance of a "plump" baby are intimately tied to a mother's feelings of satisfaction and accomplishment.

A more informed mother will realize that avoiding overfeeding and maintaining an accurate balance of food intake versus energy needs for growth will serve the child better in the long haul. Health care providers are alerted now to the dangers of overweight in early infancy, and can assist parents in monitoring the optimal growth of the infant.

MYTH BUSTER:

The most common cause of excessive early weight gain is feeding more calories than the baby actually needs to grow. Martin Stein, M.D., author of "Encounters with Children" says: "One example is a mother who was breastfeeding every time the baby cried (every 2 hours) for 12 feedings per day, each lasting 10–20 minutes. The situation was corrected when the mother understood that some babies have a great need to suck, even though they are not 'hungry'. So she experimented with alternative ways to quiet the baby, including the use of a pacifier. Another bottle-fed baby was getting 40–45 ounces of formula/day — well over the recommended 32 ounces per day. This overfeeding pattern was corrected by the same techniques mentioned above, plus replacing or diluting one bottle each day with water."

Sometimes, babies fall off the curve of a steady gradual increase in weight. This can signal a maternal depression, which is not that uncommon. Mothers may have excessive tiredness, yet be unable to sleep, and have feelings of sadness, lack of energy and hopelessness, which may result in inability to give adequate childcare. This in turn may cause infant feeding problems, resulting in feeding either too much or not enough. Nowadays this problem, called postpartum depression, is recognizable and treatable, so do not be put off by imagined stigma but get help.

Temperament

Early on, at least by 3 months of age, you can begin to detect elements of your child's personality. As you become aware of how this particular child is unique, it will provide clues as to what to expect in terms of parenting tasks, and preventing your child from becoming overweight.

An **"easy child"** (wish that each family could get at least one of these!) is characterized by a rather matter-of fact temperament that results in a general overall positive mood, average level of activity, regular sleep patterns and easily adaptable manner, among other things. The difficult to soothe, very active baby, also jokingly known as a **"mother-killer,"** will display a negative mood, over-activity, large response to stimulus, and increased motor activity level. The **"quiet,"** withdrawn or shy child may be "slow to warm up" or may seem to be the "perfect baby" who just eats and sleeps.

One of these temperamental characteristics relates to motor activity. Some infants move around a lot, others lie quietly. All infants will go through cycles of being alert and moving their arms and legs. They need this "wriggle room" to begin to explore their environment. Even babies from 1-4 months of age need baby exercise: tummy time on the floor for development of muscles, head and neck control, and encouraging activity and movement.

Can't something be done about the **crying**, doctor? Crying is a form of "exercise" that is quite normal for babies. In the first 3 months of life babies normally cry and are irritable, typically beginning in the early evening. This can last 2–3 hours per day at age 6 weeks and then decrease to an hour a day by 3 months.

This is normal behavior for this age range, and should not be confused with the need for food, especially if adequate feeding has occurred, diapers are changed, and no obvious source of discomfort is noted.

Although they are normal, these crying bouts are very disconcerting to parents. Rocking and swaddling techniques have proven to be helpful for these extended crying bouts. Avoid over-stimulating the baby after a late night feed. You are hoping quiet and swaddling will result in sleeping through the night.

Kristen Copeland, M.D., suggests: "Try dancing/moving to music with your colicky baby."

Exploration, reaching for objects, grabbing blocks, rattles, adult-assisted "walking" (with the adult holding both the baby's hands), peek-a-boo, smiling and crawling are great fun for both parent and child. The enjoyment a baby gets from exertion and learning motor skills is a wonder to behold, and helps burn calories as well.

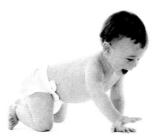

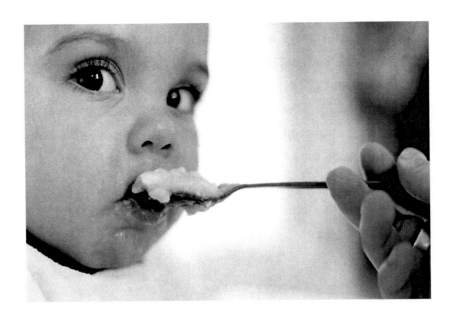

10

MISCONCEPTION:
Baby's First Foods Are Not:
Easy, Convenient,
Tasty and Cheap

Ever heard this? "What that baby needs is some stick-to-the-ribs food!"

"I really don't know when to start him on solid foods."

"I think he would sleep longer with more food in him."

REALITY CHECK:

Believe it or not, babies can do very well on breast milk alone up to 6 months of age!

There are a few signs to watch for to help you decide when to start solid foods. When babies nurse, or are offered the bottle, the mother may notice "tongue thrusting" — a response of pushing out what is placed at the entrance to the mouth. This is a reflex that tends to disappear as the child gets older. It is wise to not start trying to introduce solid foods (e.g. cereals, baby food) while the baby still has an active tongue thrust reflex.

Other indicators to look for before introducing solid food and self-feeding include the physical ability to sit up steadily, and to reach for and hold a cup or spoon.

MYTH BUSTER:

Some studies have suggested that introducing solid foods too early may influence the development of obesity in later childhood. Whether this is related more to a pattern of overfeeding with more calories than is really required for normal growth or is rather something intrinsic in the nature of the solid food is not known.

Here is an easy way to introduce solid foods, without buying a lot of extra calories such as sugars that are often included in prepared baby "first foods." There are also other benefits of preparing your baby's first foods yourself: no preservatives, freshly prepared, better vitamins and nutrients, no additives.

Here's what to do. Try steaming extra fruit or vegetables. Puree or blend them. Do not add salt or corn sugar. Babies don't need the extra flavoring. Pour the puree into ice cube trays: each one makes a perfect size serving for the baby. How easy is that?

MYTH BUSTER:

The average baby in the United States will consume 600 jars of baby food. Why is sugar added? Because Mom tastes it. Parents who use processed baby food spend an average of $300 or more on baby food during their infant's first year of life. Making baby food at home is extremely cost-effective.

Kristen Copeland, M.D. says: "If you are a working Mom and don't have time to prepare baby's first foods, don't feel too guilty. Both my very skinny girls got the purchased baby food with the sugar. I was glad to have it there, because both were pretty picky eaters when it came to anything but breast-milk."

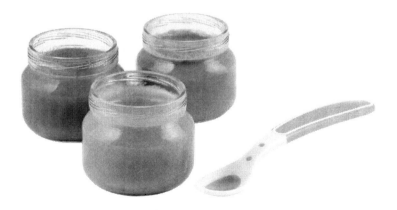

Introducing Solid Foods

Age	Additional Nutrient Need	Types of Food	Other Examples of Food	Amount
Birth to 6 Months	Exclusive breast milk or forumla	None		
5 to 7 Months	Iron	Iron-fortified rice baby ceral. Rice cereal is the least allergenic grain product	Ripe mashed avacado. Ripe mashed banana. Cooked pureed sweet potato.	Breastfeeding 5 times a day, or 32 ounces of formula bottles or breast-feeding. Solid food: 1 or 2 food servings* once in the morning and once in the afternoon.
6 to 8 Months	Vitimins A and C; variety in the diet	Vegetables such as asparagus, carrots, green beans, peas and summer squash, pureed or mashed. Then fruits such as papaya, pears, apples, and peaches, pureed or mashed. Note: Start with vegetables. If sweet fruit is introduced first, then a child may reject vegetables	Wholegrain cereal: oats, millet, brown rice. Cottage cheese Yogurt Hard-cooked egg yolk	Breastfeeding 5 times a day, or 30-32 ounces of formula or breast-feeding. Solid food: 2 to 3 food servings* morning, lunch and evening
7 to 10 Months	B Vitamins	Finger foods such as breads (e.g. crackers) and cereal (Toasted O's) Lumpy fruits and vegetables. 100% fruit juice in cup	Natural cheeses, cubed Broccoli, Plums, Watermellon, Apple	Breastfeeding at least 3 times a day or 24-32 ounces of formula. Solid food: 3 food serv-ings* morning, lunch and evening plus two snacks
8 to 12 Months	Protein: Trace Elements	Soft and cooked table foods. Ground or finely diced meats	Legumes: lentils & baked beans. Red Meat, Iron fortified breakfast cereals, Bread	Same as above. May add 2 to 4 ounces of juice

* 1 Serving = 1-2 tablespoons

64

"My baby just doesn't eat like she used to."

Between infancy and 2 years, relative nutritional need actually decreases, because the rate of both height and weight gain incrementally decreases from birth to 2 years. The active 1-year-old needs about 5–6 small meals a day. (This wouldn't be a bad idea for us all, but usually our adult schedules will not allow for it.) Again, you decide the kinds of healthy foods to offer, and let the infant and young child decide how much. Youngsters have a built-in capacity to regulate the amount of food intake they need.

Play is the key idea for the major developmental tasks during this age period. Food is included in this! Children will developmentally need to play with their food, and as they are learning to manage the switch from being fed to eating on their own, much "fall-out" is likely to occur.

"There is as much fall-out on the baby and on the floor as went down the hatch!"

Similarly, learning to navigate and get around physically requires a safe "environment." Put away those easily breakable family heirlooms and keepsakes for a while. Make sure that stairs and high places are appropriately gated.

A young toddler knows no fear, so adequate support along with vigilance toward unknown dangers such as sleeping dogs, hot pots and busy streets are in order.

Between birth and two, almost no justified "punishment" is required. However, the parent must scan the environment for safety and remove or distract the child from potentially hazardous situations. Curiosity and learning are fueled by play. A good source of distraction is looking at a picture book with bright colors. Crawling, walking and reaching are all motor skills that can be encouraged by parents, rather than seeing them as potentially dangerous.

They say we often raise our children the way we were raised! **Try to recall the way you were raised — harshly or easily, no guidance or too many rules — and pick the things that you want to carry on now in your own family and those that you want to change.**

Very short "time- outs" work well from ages 2 onward. There is never a need to hit, or slap a child's hand at any time. Considering some of these things now, early in your child's development, will help you make decisions later.

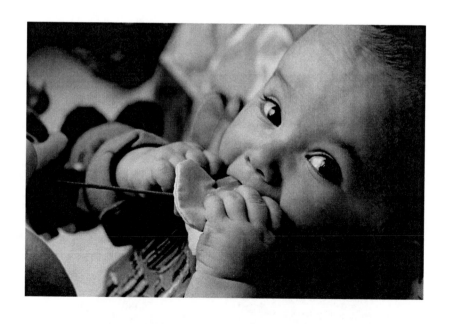

See Chapter 24 for a summary of Do's and Don'ts for Infancy

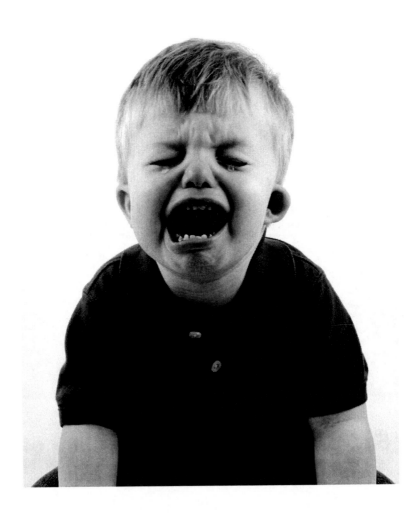

11

MYTH:
The Myth of "No!"

Ever heard this? "No! I don' wanna!"

"Aw, come on honey, just one more bite."

"No ice cream if you don't eat your carrots!"

REALITY CHECK:

Terrible Twos

This age gets a bad rap because of the assertion of independence and control that the child is beginning to exert. Two-year-olds often say "no" because they hear this word so often: Moms and Dads tell the child "no" as they reach for something hot, try to walk off the porch, or take a toy that they want. Instead of saying "no" out loud, pick the child up, remove the "danger," and redirect their attention to another activity or toy.

One way two-year-olds show their independence is in wanting to feed themselves, control you and their intake of food, or smear and play with their food. The best strategy for avoiding these battles is to give choices rather than say no to everything. Have a sense of humor and build up your resistance to seeing messes — they can be cleaned up and this stage won't last forever.

The preschooler is the center of his or her universe. Preschoolers also want and demand "to do it myself." This may take some patience on the part of the parent and willingness to see a T-shirt on backwards, or shoes untied, without a "little" assistance.

Are you tired of seeing your child eat cereal with milk for breakfast, lunch and dinner? Rather than pulling your hair out, work with her independence by trying this strategy: Pull out two (this is the magic number) kinds of cereal for breakfast. Allow her to make the decision of which kind she'll eat. Make a big deal about what a "big" girl she is. This way you are rewarding the behavior you previously were fighting against. At lunch, try giving her a choice of a peanut butter sandwich on whole wheat bread, or cheese and crackers. Hopefully, she'll be so thrilled with the opportunity to choose that she'll forget about her cereal and milk rut. If she insists on cereal, try, try again until you guide her away from the cereal and milk.

Preschoolers will grow about 2½ inches per year and gain about 4½ pounds per year. The rate of growth continues to decline after the first year of life, and leads you to notice a decreased appetite. It's normal.

The types of foods that children and adults need are the same. The difference is that children should be fed child-size portions only. **A common cause of overfeeding in this age group is serving adult-sized portions to young children.** The average serving size for toddlers is small: about the same as the size of their fist!

Veggies, fruits: 1–1½ cups; grains 3–5 ounces; meat 1–2 ounces; milk 2 cups — all for a 24-hour period.

The best strategy is this: start regular meal times by putting food on the table. Help serve or allow kids to help themselves put the amount on their plate they think they want.

Encourage taking a little bit of everything, but allow a child to limit something they don't really like that much. **And don't make a fuss over eating!** If kids don't eat what is on their plate, try smaller serving sizes. **Don't insist on "cleaning the plate."**

If you worry that they are not eating enough: watch their growth patterns. If they are growing normally and not putting on extra weight, you are doing exactly what you should as a caring parent!

Take a look at how balanced your family's diet is:

- Are there plenty of fruits and vegetables to get the recommended five servings per day?

- Do you use fat to cook? If so, what kind?

- How many sugary snacks do you have available in the house? The best thing to do is have sweet foods available and offer them every once in a while. If you never offer them, your child will go crazy at preschool or birthday parties (much like adults when we've denied our sweet tooth).

Research shows that eating together as a family is not only a positive social experience: a family who dines together at home eats more fruits and vegetables, less sugar and fat, less soda and less calories.

MYTH BUSTER:

There is no need for children over one year of age to have whole milk. Watch out for the "trained night feeder", too much milk consumption (even one percent fat) adds calories and inhibits iron absorption possibly causing iron deficiency anemia. If you are concerned, check with your doctor.

MYTH BUSTER:

Just as adults rarely eat while they are sleeping, there is no need for a child to take a bottle to bed for nourishment or soothing purposes. Kathy Kaufer Christoffel, M.D., says: "I remember the 3-year-old referred to my weight clinic who was clutching the bottle and the history showed going to bed with the bottle ... it was so easy to see what changes were needed."

Preschool children are tremendously curious, but cannot distinguish between reality and fantasy. Hence, this is the age of magic, of imaginary playmates and the dastardly deeds of the family cat or dog (such as knocking over Mom's favorite flower vase).

This high degree of imagination and lack of distinction between reality and fantasy makes preschoolers easy targets for television advertisements featuring appealing cartoon characters. These characters are easily recognized by the preschooler, who will point them out to Mom on a cereal box at the supermarket. The advertised character may also lead to a request to stop at a fast food establishment to obtain a toy or cup.

Parents should be aware of this influence, and not give in to the child's unrelenting requests to get a toy and compromise their nutritional needs.

How parents treat the toddler's imagination can plant the seeds for obesity

Response of parents to the imaginary and "story telling" behaviors of their toddler can reinforce either a sense of satisfaction and growth, or a sense of shame and guilt. All children want is to please their parents and receive praise. A sensitive response to a "golly-wobble" (as my grandmother dubbed it) shows acceptance of the child while at the same time recognizing the fun and fantasy aspects of the "tall tale." Direct parental criticism to what the child did, not to the child: "I didn't like the way you behaved" rather than "You are so bad."

The growing sense of autonomy during this period may challenge a parent who wants to "control" and govern the range of behaviors and emotions that their child displays. Sensitivity to the child's temperamental characteristics will help the parent avoid confrontations that only result in somebody losing (usually the child). **Distraction and redirection of interests work better than opposition to the child's desires at the age of 2 to 3 years.**

We learn to give attention for "bad" behavior rather than "good" behavior. A good alternative strategy is to watch for behavior you like and give lots of attention and praise when it happens. You will find that "good" behavior increases!

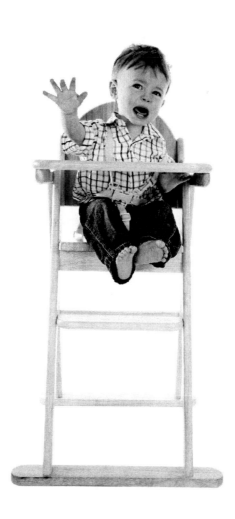

12

MYTH:
Toddlers Should Be
Seen And Not Heard

Ever heard this? "Will you please stop screaming?"
"Stop running around — you'll fall!"
"Sit down, be quiet, and watch this TV
show!"

REALITY CHECK:

The desire to move around, jump, play games, run, hide and
be active with siblings, peers, parents, grandparents and
other family members seems to be well established in almost
all children. **The key to having an active preschooler is to
provide plenty of opportunities for active play, preferably
outside, that are safe.** In other words, just let play happen
and make opportunities available, and most children will be
active.

Play is so much more than, well, just playing.

REMEMBER

P = Provide opportunities for kids to play

L = Link play with fun, and activity will come naturally

A = Actively seek activities your kids enjoy

Y = You participate, too!

Toddlers need to have the opportunities to do things over and over in order to learn new skills and do them well. Also, play is about exploring their world, what their bodies are capable of and discovering their own sense of their body, their creativity and their imaginations. The more your toddler plays, the better sleep they will get and the more likely they will maintain a healthy weight.

At this age, favorite toys and activities include:

- Toys that look like adult tools such as a lawn mower, kitchen appliances, shopping cart, rake or broom. Toddlers like to copy parents doing things.

- Toys they can push or pull.

- Large and light balls to repeat movements such as throwing or rolling the ball over and over again.

- Blocks to dump out of their container.

- Ride-on toys your child can push with the feet, or a tricycle to pedal.

None of these activities require a fancy toy or gyms. In fact, haven't you ever noticed your child is happier playing with the box and wrapping paper than the toy that was in the box to begin with?

Other household items your toddler would love to play with (if you haven't guessed already):

- Plastic and metal bowls
- Plastic measuring spoons and cups
- Pots and pans
- Wooden spoons
- Oatmeal box
- Pillows

Favorite games of toddlers include:

- Dancing to music
- Follow-the-leader
- Hide-and-seek
- Make believe cooking, or cleaning the house or yard
- Chase me (picture a child running with glee, being pursued by grandparent/adult)

It is a mystery to most adults why a child of this age never tires of being "chased," caught or almost caught, and released to flee again with screams of delight. I have never seen a child terminate a play episode of "chase me," but I've seen many adults! If you have a preschooler, this game will help them get their needed activity, and help you burn off a few extra calories yourself. Watch out for uneven turf, but even a spill on the grass is usually quickly forgotten, and the only residue is a grass stain on the trousers!

Research studies have shown that active children tend to get rated by parents as more aggressive, loud and disruptive than less active children, so watch comments that discourage activity. Prompts from adults and peers to be active are one of the strongest determinants of the activity levels of preschool children, so long as there is a place for them to be active. Interestingly, prompts not to be active are equally effective. So watch out for too many comments such as "sit down," "be quiet," and "be careful," when the time is right for active play.

It is not until later that children begin to learn from adults and others to "sit down," "be quiet," and "stop running around." Observe the temperament of your child to see if they will need some extra encouragement to be active with others. For example, a shy child may need to have protected "play dates" with only one other child when fun things like chase and tag can be part of the play.

The main task of parents is to make sure there are safe places to play both at home and in the neighborhood, or at day care arrangements. Safety also includes supervision or at least eye-sight line of vision monitoring in an already determined physically safe area. Children vary in their coordination, ability to throw, kick and catch a ball, but all get great pleasure from "playing." Be careful not to play the "coach and teacher" too much.

GAMES TEACH SKILLS

Tag, the well-known game that is a favorite of all, teaches agility, speed, rapid starting and stopping, changing direction, eye–hand coordination and body movements to avoid the "tag," as well as fun interaction with a buddy or the "it" person.

Throwing/Catching teaches eye–hand coordination in catching the ball, arm and body strength in throwing, and accuracy in direction of throw. The younger the child, the larger, lighter and softer the ball. Two-handed throwing is an easier first step than one-handed throwing. Don't forget you also get a pretty good workout chasing after the ball!

Kicking works on eye–foot coordination, lower limb strength and coordination (if running and kicking). Again, a bigger ball is easier to spot, and softer ones are better suited for the toddler. It is also better for the ball to be kicked rather than the little brother or the family dog!

Skipping Rope. This activity is almost the property of young school age girls, but for boys who can imagine themselves as professional boxers, it is a great activity to build aerobic capacity, coordination and whole body fitness. It is great with music or chanting rhymes. "Other benefits of jumping rope include improved timing, rhythm, agility, bone density and quickness. I think it's important for children to participate in some group activities as these can be useful for learning basic social skills and can lead to the development of friendships." –Tim Haft, Trainer.

Hop Scotch. Another common activity that builds skills in moving the entire body in space according to a planned direction. I have seen both boys and girls enjoy this activity on a neighborhood sidewalk.

Tumbling. Who hasn't seen kids roll down a hill, turn somersaults, and attempt to stand on their heads? These are early "play" forms of tumbling and gymnastics.

Puppy "Wrestling" (example courtesy of Tim Haft, Trainer). Picture a batch of new puppies. They are all over each other, "wrestling" and then napping! This is nature's way of conditioning them to the interactions they will have with other dogs when they grow up. There is never an intent to harm another puppy. What would happen if human "pups" had a similar opportunity? It might result in kids not being afraid to touch or be touched and have close interactions with others. They would also learn how to play without intending to harm another person. If children were permitted this type of rough and tumble play, it might influence how they interact with others when they grow up. Instead, we are very concerned that if siblings or boys are "tussling" someone might get hurt or cry — and the adult peace-keeper and police officer will intervene. If this is done to excess, then kids may never get exposed to the rough and tumble aspects of contact play, and hence will be afraid of it as harmful to themselves or others, or displeasing to adults.

Swimming. While teaching young children to swim and feel comfortable in the water is a good idea, it is impossible to "drown proof" a young child! Whenever children are in the water an adult (parent) needs to be at arms length. Home pools of all types need to be secured behind locked fences. A young child, if they fall into the water will sink. Parents should play with their kids and help them with swimming skills, but let formal instruction be done by trained teachers.

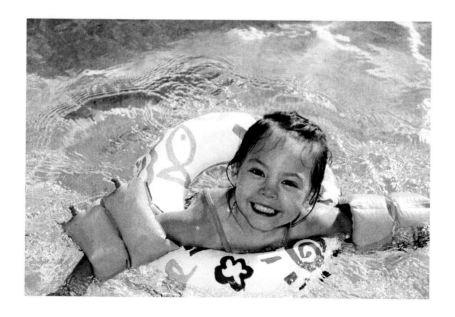

13

MISCONCEPTION:
Day Care and TV Mind Your
Kids And Have Your Child's
Best Interests At Heart!

Ever heard this? "There's not that much difference
between day care sites."
"My kids just love children's TV. It would
be bad to limit it."

REALITY CHECK:

There is no parent, grandparent or baby-sitter alive who hasn't
used the television set at times as a convenient way to distract,
quiet down, and manage kids. Similarly, out-of-home day care
is a reality for the working mother and "dual income" family.

For both of these realities the trick is to:

- Know how much screen time is appropriate.
- Realize that all day care is not created equal.

Picture a TV set saying: "Let me watch your kids, keep them quiet, and sell them sugary foods."

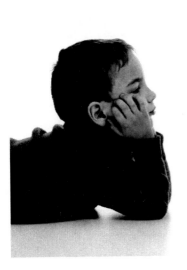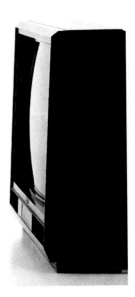

There are many worthwhile TV programs and learning with entertainment available for children. One of the leading children's daytime TV shows has recently "gone dark" during the day for selected periods in order to encourage parents to take their child outside to play!

MYTH BUSTER:

As well as the association between hours of TV watched and overweight (high BMI), there are the added impacts of the effects of TV advertisements influencing children to request certain food and toy items. Young children can recognize brands and logos. Children who watch aggressive behavior on TV are more likely to engage in aggressive behavior themselves, and there are many acts of violence on TV every week. There are a growing number of households with television sets in each child's room, and many households that allow or encourage eating in front of the TV for both adults and children alike.

There is a large discrepancy between the 1–2 hours a day of supervised TV viewing time recommended by the Academy of Pediatrics and the 3–7 hours a day the average TV in the United States is turned on! Parents will have to take an active role in setting reasonable limits on TV viewing.

Tom Robinson, M.D., Stanford University: "It is the one thing [TV viewing] that when experimentally reduced has been effective in decreasing weight gain among children." Tom has also done a recent study showing that 3–5 year old children say that foods (even carrots) wrapped in McDonald's paper taste better than identical foods wrapped in plain paper! For information on the school-based curriculum for reduction of might have a protective effect over time for most kids. Limit it to 1–2 hours, remove TVs from bedrooms, and avoid eating while watching TV. **A good tip for prevention: Don't put a TV in a child's bedroom! It is very difficult to get it out once it is in there!**

"Health-Proofing" the Day Care Environment You Choose for Your Child

Regardless of the amount of hours per day that a child spends in day care or preschool facilities, parents need to know a lot about the quality of that environment.

Do you know the timing and nature of meals served at the center, as well as the opportunities for active play? Teachers and aides who are well versed in principles of child development are more likely to be the norm in larger centers, but in smaller or home-centered care there may be more variability.

As well as observing the educational and child-development orientation of the school or day care facility, give equal consideration to opportunities for safe, active play and availability of nutritious food. Observe a prospective day care center or preschool before enrolling your child. Spot observations are a good idea during the year, especially if there is a change in leadership or ownership of the facility.

Things to investigate in choosing a day care center

- What are the food preparation facilities?
- How are menus planned, if snacks or meals are provided?
- What are the food safety provisions?
- When are snacks served?
- What is the variety and nature of the snacks provided?
- Is play equipment safe?
- Is it appropriate to the age and skill levels of the children?
- Are play surfaces grass or soft?
- Are artificial surfaces soft and resilient?
- Is there a danger of falling from a tall structure onto a concrete or stone pavement?
- Does the facility offer both structured and unstructured playtime?
- Is outdoor activity emphasized?
- What happens during inclement weather with regard to active play?
- Is a television a part of the program at any time?
- How and when is it used?
- What are arrangements for napping if required?
- How many children per adult teacher or aide?

MYTH BUSTER:

What are the size of the groups that eat together at day care? For adults, the larger the group the more "socializing" takes place, and the more food people eat — and the same holds for kids. What about fruits and vegetables as opposed to cakes and cookies?

By taking into account the same standards you want to provide at home for your child, you will assure that the day care or preschool environment is supporting your efforts, not undermining them.

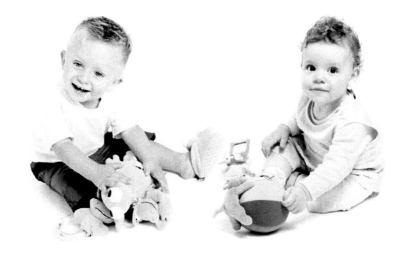

14

MISCONCEPTION:
At Age Three, Nothing Can Be Done To Prevent Obesity

Ever heard this? "My child demands candy and chips."

"I love sweets myself, how can I deprive her?"

"My grandmother always had a sweet for me."

"If you clean up your plate you can have some candy."

REALITY CHECK:

We did a study of over 1,000 children in 10 locations around the United States. If a preschool child's weight went over the 85th percentile only one time, they had a five times greater risk of being overweight by age 12 years. What was even more surprising was that the level that made a 3-year-old girl of average height "overweight" (at or above the 85th percentile) was **only four pounds!**

To remind you, here are the amounts of extra weight a child has to put on at different ages in order to get to levels that the CDC says are either "overweight" or actually "obese."

Age	Normal weight in pounds	Extra pounds to to be overweight	Extra pounds to be obese
3	32	+4 = 36	+6 = 38
7	55	+3 = 58	+ 10 = 65
12	104	+15 = 119	+ 34 = 138

Now, suppose you check out your toddler on the CDC BMI charts (http://cdc.gov/nccdphp/dnpa/bmi/index.htm), and find that he or she is overweight or obese. You will of course check with your health care provider.

However, don't be surprised if there is not much of a reaction or concern. After all, what parent or doctor would get excited about a 3-year-old who is only 4 pounds over normal?

But if we don't act early when this adding on of extra weight starts, we start losing the battle against preventing obesity! Remember, this does not call for a diet, only an awareness of the types and amounts of food eaten and opportunities for activity. Many times, the main causes of even a few extra pounds are habits of eating lots of candy, sweets, or cakes, or watching TV inside instead of going outside to play.

You can be a detective to make sure:

- There is a good variety of healthy foods and snacks available.

- Excessive sweets and fats are limited.

- Portion size is appropriate to a preschooler.

- There is outside activity at least an hour a day.

- TV time is limited to 1–2 hours a day.

Tips on Healthy Toddler Snacks

- Don't carry food around to offer if child is bored or fussy, offer snacks only when child indicates hunger.

- Cut up slices of vegetables and fruit (just a quarter of a cup will do) and place them in plastic bags in the refrigerator.

- Be careful that your child doesn't drink a lot of fruit juice, which adds up to a significant amount of calories.

- Almost any "real food" or food in its natural, unprocessed state is preferable to a bag of chips, candy, or packaged cookie or cake.

Life is sweet — What's a treat?

Children and adults vary in their affinity and desire for sweets. This could be due to genetics or early experience. Some can take it or leave it, others drive cars with license plate holders that read, "Hand over the chocolate and no one gets hurt." The consumption of sweets is almost always associated with pleasant or stimulating events such as parties, or extra attention from adults and friends. The "strong sweet tooth" is most likely a learned and reinforced habit. When adults are stressed, sales of sugar and sweets increase.

While the authors do not recommend a "scrooge-like" approach to birthdays, holidays and Halloween, try to emphasize the event and not the excessive consumption of sugar, fat and candy. Of course have some birthday cake and ice cream! Of course enjoy the costumes and "scary" images of Halloween, allow one evening of munching down on the treats, then discard the remainder.

The occasional candy binge is possibly less harmful than a child-rearing practice that permits a well-known location of a stash of candy that is available for dispensing by the parent as a reward, or even available on demand by the child. A quick trip to the "candy drawer" can be a great solace to a child who is lonely at home after school, or merely bored.

The solution: Don't have a "candy stash drawer" for either the kids or the grown-ups! But do have easily available healthy snacks.

"Eat all your supper and you can have some candy." Not only does this teach the child not to respond appropriately to body signals of feeling full, but if they comply, they put in more calories than their body needs, by getting the reward with its extra calories. Another "bonus" is that candy (particularly the sticky kind or lots of raisins), can potentially damage teeth. Even cavities in baby teeth can affect the health of your child's adult teeth.

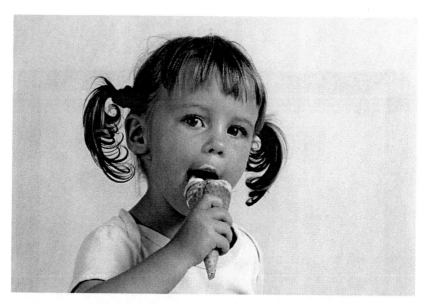

See Chapter 24 For A Summary of Do's and Don'ts for Preschoolers.

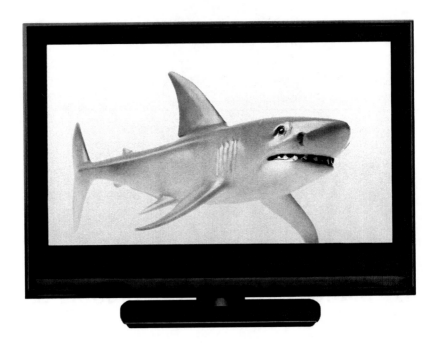

15

MISCONCEPTION:
Parents Have More to Fear from Strangers Kidnapping their Kid than from Business and Marketing

Ever heard this? "Stay where I can see you."
                        "Don't talk to strangers."

REALITY CHECK:

There is nothing wrong with these admonitions, although most child abduction is carried out by family members or people the child knows. But with what level of vigor do we also try to protect our kids from the $30 billion market directed towards children ages 5–17? Kids could see 50,000 TV commercials each year, and many of these undermine our attempts to have kids eat healthy food and be more active.

Forty percent of parents of school age children are afraid of their child being kidnapped. Compare this to 9 million children over age 6 who are obese; and the 30–50% of children in some neighborhoods who are already obese by school entry. We need to be as vigilant in protecting our kids from marketing as we are about child abduction.

The effects of marketing don't stop there. Food is marketed differently to rich and to poor neighborhoods. This tends to worsen the higher rates of obesity in children who reside in economically distressed neighborhoods. This translates into more fast food outlets and fewer supermarkets in poor neighborhoods. A recent Institute of Medicine Report analyzed the cost of fresh fruits and vegetables and determined that the cost would be within the reach of low-income families. But many families today do not have enough money. Both access and price need to be addressed.

Research: When supermarkets were made more accessible in a low-income area, African Americans in one study increased their consumption of vegetables by 20%.

It doesn't stop with food. Parents' fears about allowing their children to go roam away from home to pursue their independent play and exploration has led to a noticeable drop in sales of 20-inch bikes (the size for children aged 8–10 years) since 1987. **Phil Nader, M.D., says: "When I was growing up, I would leave home on my bike on a Saturday morning, taking a sandwich, and return by suppertime. The spirit of adventure and self-confidence was very exciting, and it was quite safe from the point of view of traffic and crime."**

Today, it might not be advisable to allow your child to do this, but we need to come up with alternative ways to replace some of the natural burning of energy along with the fostering of independence that used to occur.

Statistics reveal a great change in the amount of activity children get, including getting to school and back home. Whereas 80% of children once walked to school, now 80% ride in a car or school bus. That equates to a big change in the daily expenditure of calories for our kids.

Recent new programs include a "walking" school bus, in which parents and adult volunteers take turns walking with children to and from school. These programs are along designated, well-marked and publicized routes to assure safety and visibility.

Safe bike trails could be organized for older kids. Think about organizing such a program for you and your neighbors. Being on your own on a bike ride builds confidence, a sense of adventure, and accomplishment, in addition to burning calories.

The culture of marketing fits in well with what is happening at the stage of development when children officially leave the nest, and the carefree playtime of preschool, to enter the "workaday" world of school. This is when the slippery slope of decreasing activity begins!

This is where parents begin to realize that they no longer have the only voice in what happens to their kid. **Others — both kids and adults —** now have an equal say (if not more) in influencing kids' choices about eating and activity, and also about many other life decisions. **Remember, you are still the director and producer of the film your child is starring in!**

But it does mean giving up the dictatorial role. "I am your father, and I say so," doesn't hold the clout it used to. It now becomes more and more important to be able to relate to your child with an open mind and the ability to understand their temperament and what they are feeling and thinking.

Being an "activity and food" detective is going to become more important to the adult interested in protecting kids from obesity. **In other words, you have to be aware of the big world out there with as much concern about a healthy environment as your kids' physical safety!** This may require learning new skills of activism, advocacy, and doing something about conditions you see as adverse to kids' health.

Remember, you still control the home environment. Keep up as much as possible eating family meals together even if it requires fixing and freezing on weekends!

Children do grow and gain weight during their school age years. Studies show that children who maintained a BMI at or below the 50th percentile during the preschool years rarely become overweight or obese as children and adolescents.

Have you plotted where your child is on the BMI growth chart? We have seen that an average height 7-year-old girl needs only 3 extra pounds to be overweight and only 10 extra pounds to be "obese."

Kids this age could "grow into" that amount of extra weight, by keeping with a simple 5,4,3,2,1:

- 5 servings of fruits and vegetable a day
- 4 glasses of water
- 3 low-fat dairy or meat servings
- 2 hours of screen time, and
- At least 1 hour of physical activity.

(Courtesy CLOCC — Consortium to Lower Obesity in Chicago Children www.clocc.net)

Easy snacks for kids of all ages

- Cut up fresh, raw carrots, sweet peppers, carrots and celery with low-fat ranch dressing.

- Frozen peas and carrots or frozen blueberries right out of the package

- Fresh fruit salad: cut up a banana and apple, and peel a tangerine. Mix together. Add 3 tablespoons of non-fat, plain yogurt, 1 tablespoon of honey, 1 teaspoon of vanilla. Pour over fruit. Enjoy!

- Instant banana pudding: mash ½ small banana, 3 tablespoons of unsweetened applesauce, and 1 teaspoon of non-fat plain yogurt. Eat.

- Quick fruit kabobs: cut up banana, apple, cantaloupe and low-fat cheese into cubes. Put on skewer. Dip in orange juice. Roll in coconut or low-fat granola. Yummy!

- Energy trail mix: put 2 tablespoons of raisins in bowl, and 1 teaspoon each of unsalted, shelled peanuts, sunflower seeds, coconut, carob or chocolate chips. Mix.

- Smiley toast: toast a slice of whole-wheat bread. Spread 1 tablespoon of natural peanut butter. Use three slices of banana (two for eyes, one for nose) and raisins for a smile.

- Quick and simple: fresh fruits and vegetables, non-fat yogurt, graham crackers, pretzels, microwave low-fat popcorn, sorbet, sherbet, non-fat frozen yogurt.

Kids also enjoy making their own snacks and kid snack recipe books are out there!

How to handle holidays and celebrations without going overboard.

Halloween

- Go trick or treating. Allow your child to eat as much as they want that night or the next day. Throw the rest away. Or store in the freezer. Bring out for the occasional treat.

Thanksgiving or Winter Holidays

- Plan a physical activity before the eating begins. I know of one family who plays an annual touch football game with team T-shirts on Thanksgiving. Go on a walk.

- Have fresh, cut-up fruits and veggies that people can fill up on instead of just the fattening foods.

- Make sure water is available and not just apple juice or eggnog.

- Offer smaller plates. People, including children, will eat less.

- Use smaller serving utensils. That way people can't serve as much.

- Start off with a salad.

Valentine's Day

- Make homemade Valentine cards with your child for her class … instead of cupcakes.

- Have a pink–red themed party. Serve red fruit, such as strawberries, raspberries, and red apples. Serve red veggies, such as red peppers, tomatoes and radishes with low-fat ranch dressing with a drop of red food coloring mixed in.

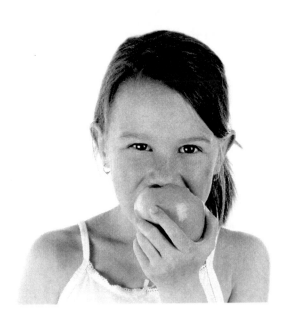

16

MYTH:
They Will Get Lots of Activity and Healthy Food at School and After School Programs

Ever heard this? "We used to have recess and PE every day, don't you?"
"We couldn't buy soda pop at school when I was a kid."

REALITY CHECK:

There is no doubt that, across the country, both the amount and quality of school PE has decreased in recent years, perhaps because of the increased emphasis on basic academics. Some data suggests that schools that have better quality PE programs also have better scores on academics.

A huge amount of a child's nutrition comes from school nutrition programs in this country. It starts with breakfast and lunch, and continues in many places with before and after school programs.

The USDA, which administers school lunch and breakfast programs and controls food subsidies for schools, recently required all schools to have a "wellness" plan or policy, and food and nutrition guidelines that are supposed to limit unhealthy choices and foster healthy ones for kids. Check to see if your child's school has such a policy. If the school does, *is it being implemented?*

We did a study of the amount and quality of structured physical education classes for over 1,000 third grade children in 10 different sites in the United States. Fewer than 6% of children had daily PE in school. They generally had two classes per week of about 33 minutes each. Of this time in PE, about 25 minutes per lesson was spent in moderate to vigorous physical activity. This is far short of national recommendations for at least an hour a day of physical activity. In addition, many schools no longer have recess periods, and those that do lack the environment (e.g. no balls to play with) or the support (no aides on the playground to encourage physical activity) for kids to be active during that time.

Now is the time to find out about the school that your child attends.

How often do they have PE and what is the quality of that PE? What are school lunches like? Are there salad bars and fresh vegetables? What about sales of snack foods, and money-raising events for school clubs or teams?

How vigilant are school principals and teachers about making sure that treats are healthy rather than empty calories such as candy?

More and more schools are sporting school gardens, salad bars, and lower fat entrees, but we still have many schools with vending machines selling candy and soda drinks. Pouring and vending contracts have been a source of much-needed funds for schools, but the quantities sold have resulted in some states passing laws to ban soda drink sales in schools.

The only way to know what your child's school is like is to visit the school, and inquire about it.

Your child spends more time at school than almost anywhere else. Hopefully you can help make sure that time is not spent in an environment of poor nutrition and lack of physical activity.

MYTH BUSTER:

What is active PE? You can tell a quality PE program by watching the kids. Is everyone moving, or are they taking turns, standing around, lining up, etc.? Take a moment some day to find out the schedule of PE in your child's school, and go visit. Watch out for schools that make up their mandated number of hours of PE by bunching them all together every other week with very large classes! The larger the PE class, the less activity any one child gets.

RESEARCH

The authors and others developed two current "best practice" programs that were funded by your tax dollars and the National Institutes of Health: the CATCH PE (Coordinated Approach to Child Health) is one well-studied model; and the SPARK (Sports, Physical Activity and Recreation for Kids) program, based upon the same principles as CATCH, is also well studied and broadly implemented.

The key to the success of both of these programs is continued teacher training. CATCH also has a classroom, cafeteria, and family component, and has been shown to limit the rate of weight gain among elementary school children in El Paso, Texas.

Classroom Birthday Parties

- Bring in a tray of fruit, a veggie platter, and water. Go ahead and have cupcakes, too. But bring the mini versions.

- Help your child's teacher come up with a monthly celebration. Then celebrate all the birthdays and holidays for that month at once. This cuts down on the number of parties ... and cupcakes your child consumes.

- Forego birthday celebrations with food. How about buying a book for your school's library in honor of your child?

- Consider other activities instead of eating to celebrate your child's birthday. Go outside and play a game. Another idea is to have the children in your child's class write down five things they like about your child, and then tell her.

Unsupervised time and kids spending money — peer influences and the neighborhood store.

Welcome to the world where you have very little direct control over what your child decides to do with their money! This is, in a real sense, the beginning of parenting by example and reason rather than fiat and rules!

If a child spends all their money on a candy treat, or getting similar treats for their friends to "win" their friendship, they will learn — perhaps through discussions with you — the consequences of being "broke" for the moment, or how true friendship is not sustained by superficial acts. There are more effective ways of "being a friend." Remember, the occasional sweet and empty calorie snack, if it has become contraband, only becomes more desirable!

If excessively unhealthy patterns keep being disclosed in conversations with your child, then a private visit to the storekeeper to enlist help in redirecting interest in healthy snacks might be considered. What's the availability of healthy snacks at the store anyway? How are they displayed — in end caps of aisles, etc.? Where is water displayed and is it as affordable as sodas? (More detective work!)

> ## MYTH BUSTER:
> Society has created **the child consumer.** This means that kids need to know not only about money, but how to spend it, especially when you are not around.

Here are some examples of healthy snacks vs. junk food. Both are available for purchase. The best way is to lead by example and habit!

- Bagels instead of donuts and pastries.
- Veggie pizza slice instead of pepperoni pizza slice.
- Almost anything fresh rather than something in a package.
- Fig bars or vanilla wafers instead of chocolate chip cookies.

- Baked chips, pretzels or plain popcorn instead of fried potato chips.

If you have gotten your kids used to enjoying the taste of healthy foods at an earlier age, they are much more likely to prefer the healthier varieties of so-called fast food. If you have had a reasonable balance of healthy and occasional fast food, then there is a high likelihood that this balance will not be thrown too far out with independent choices made by the child.

Here is the time when a child can gain control, exert their independence, and go along with the crowd. One issue is how much money is a child permitted to carry, and what period of time elapses between the time school is out and the child returns to a supervised environment? Reasonable amounts can be decided upon ahead of time, so that at least large quantities of candy bars etc. cannot be purchased at one time.

Know the neighborhood stores and convenience shops, know the routes home or favorite spots for the kids to hang out. Know what kind of choices they offer. It is possible to get a nutritious meal after school, and sometimes that big hunger is too large to wait until dinner!

Allowances and Spending Money

Maybe not in kindergarten or first grade, but by the time a child is in third or fourth grade and upwards, many children will have pocket change to spend as they will. However, school entry is the time when you can begin to plant the seeds of responsible spending and handling money. It can start with exercises counting the values of coins, and a piggy bank.

A prerequisite exercise for you is to think about how you manage your own money. Are you like many Americans who spend more than they have and build up impossible-to-pay-off credit card debt? If you are in this group (and you have many kindred spirits), it might be wise to get some help in straightening out your own financial picture and guidelines. Paying out an allowance of any amount — regardless of how small — is probably not a good idea until you have a good picture of how you spend your available money now.

Do kids steal? Yes!

Young children will take things — including money from Mom's purse or Dad's wallet — or lift an attractive toy from a store. This is a normal developmental event. However, the wrong must be "righted" and not ignored. Property must be returned or, if that's not possible, earned with chores or duties. Persistent stealing may also reflect some unmet emotional needs of the child, and talking with your health care provider is indicated.

If you want to instill a sense of delaying gratification and reward savings then a rather small allowance will promote these habits if there is a desired prize or attainable goal within a reasonable time period. A small goal can be achieved in a relatively short time of saving. Once the child has experienced this, then it is possible to set longer-term goals with longer time periods.

How much allowance and for what duties? How much is a relative thing for different families in different circumstances. However, it is also influenced by the current "market place" and economic trends. I continue to be amazed by the currently inflated amount the "tooth fairy" will pay for a lost tooth! I could not have fathomed getting a quarter, 50 cents or even paper money for a tooth left under the pillow when I was 6 years old!

Another consideration is what the child might be expected to buy. In my view the allowance is not to be used for routine costs such as school lunch or milk money, but rather for something the child decides upon. An allowance is just that—an allowance —that comes on a regular basis, without contingencies. Chores and household duties are considered to be the child's part in keeping up the household and contributing to the family. In turn, the family does many things to help each family member — including the allowance and other privileges. So while they are related, one does not depend upon the other.

> Laura Nathanson, M.D. says: "Remember chores can also be a great source of physical activity: taking out the garbage, sweeping, digging, washing the car, and walking the dog."

17

MISCONCEPTION:
Sexuality and Obesity
Have Nothing In Common

Ever heard this? "You're much too young to ask about
that!"

REALITY CHECK:

It used to be thought that, because young school children were
always busy and engaged in doing and learning, sexuality,
and sex-roles "disappeared" or became "latent." This could
not be further from the truth!

Just watch and listen to "boy talk" and "girl talk" about each
other in childhood! Both sexes talk about the other with
intense interest. When questions or comments are brought to
adults, sometimes the adults tend to brush off such questions
"because you are too young." What children often learn from
this is that such topics are "taboo" — just how taboo depends
upon their family and cultural environment.

Sex play ("you show me yours and I'll show you mine," and playing doctor) are part of normal development around ages 4 to 6. Matter-of-fact discussions about appropriate and not appropriate behavior can be held, along with factual and informative talks about normal anatomy and functions, without going beyond the child's level of curiosity and interest. If you are uncomfortable with these topics, there are many good books out there for parents.

MYTH BUSTER:

Children who are overweight tend to mature earlier than normal weight children. Since overweight is also associated with poor self-image, and lack of peer relationships, this could result in placing them at increased risk for early unprotected intercourse and teen pregnancy. Even if kids are not overweight, if they have a poor self-image or lack of peer relationships, they have the same risk. Another source of a lack of healthy self-image is worry or concern about other sexuality issues.

Do not wait until adolescence to become familiar with human sexuality topics and then talk to your child. Adolescence, with the raging hormones, will be too late. Your child will have already been "schooled" (and probably not well) by their peers. You need to be the best source of information and have confidential discussions with your child from early school age onwards. This open and informed approach will prepare you to be supportive to your child and help them feel valued and accepted regardless of what gender or sexuality issues may arise as they mature.

Why are we bringing up sexuality issues on a book about preventing overweight and promoting healthy lifestyles? There are connections between being overweight and sexual development. For one thing, overweight leads to earlier puberty. Part of the key to healthy development is complete acceptance and feelings of self-worth around sex.

Healthy developmental foundations are nature's way of "immunizing" kids against the detrimental effects of too early risky behaviors, depression and eating disorders. Parents who are prepared to discuss and share values associated with sexuality with their children have a complete bundle of resources to help their kids. Learn the scientific names of body parts (penis, vagina, anus) and use them properly. Answer your child's questions, but be sure you understand what it is they are asking.

Remember the story of the parent who gave a 15 minute talk on "where did I come from?" and the 5-year-old's response, after the explanation, was "Oh, I just wondered. Johnny said he was from Chicago."

You don't have to "schedule" a birds and bees talk with your young school age child, but by at least 8 years old, especially if there are any pregnant women in the child's life, expect to be asked, "Where do babies come from?" Do not put the child off by saying something like "You're too young to know that." It gives them a feeling of being demeaned and not worthy of getting an honest answer — not a good thing for a developing young ego! Instead, tell the truth.

It is better to respond in a matter-of-fact way with the whole truth, than to give incomplete answers that could lead to misconceptions.

A typical 8-year-old's response, when told exactly how babies are conceived, might be: "But my parents never did that!" Knowing the facts does not mean that they will rush out to try it.

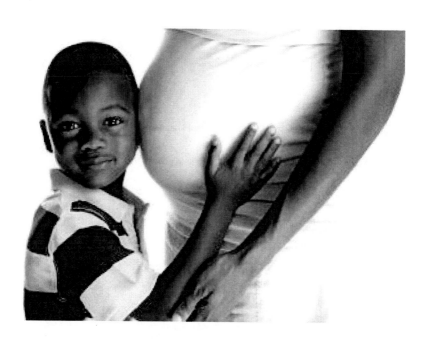

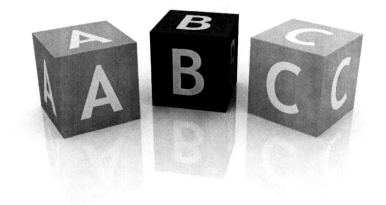

18

MISCONCEPTION: Everything in School is Fine - Don't Bother to Ask

Ever heard this?   "What did you do in school today?"
"Nothing."
"What was the best thing that happened?"
"A fight between Billy and Joey."
"What are you doing in reading?"
"Nothing."
"Do you have homework?" "Don't know."

REALITY CHECK:

School is a time for learning, and it is important to enjoy the growing accomplishments and capacities of the growing child. You can show interest in what the child says, but you may not learn everything you need to know just by talking with your child! Families and schools are always changing and it is important to keep an eye on what's happening in three areas:

- Learning
- Family and friends
- Understanding of sexual development

Why these three? Especially in a book on preventing obesity?

While the eating and activity environment are key determinants of weight gain, how a child copes with and adjusts to the stresses and rigors of life will have direct influences on their self-image, confidence in their own ability, and self-worth — all of which influence their eating habits and activity levels.

The roots of long-lasting adult problems can be traced to early school difficulties, so do not assume that school is going fine unless you hear something from the teacher. Be active in inquiring about not only academics, but also the teacher's views of your child. Ask to review your child's "cumulative folder" (a record of all school information abour your child). You have a right to remove any incorrect information you think could be harmful to your child. Pick up early on any difficulties. There are many school and healthcare professionals that you can turn to, such as school counselors and special resource teachers, nurses, psychologists and physicians.

Leaving the Nest Officially: Entering School

The "umbilical" cord pulls at both ends! Both child and parent can be anxious about starting school. The parent may have some misgivings and even perhaps feel a little threatened that another adult will begin to have influence over their child. It is best to let the child adjust to kindergarten on their own, without the presence of Mom, so a quick hug and "see you later" is the best course of action. After a few weeks you can visit or even volunteer to help if you have the time.

After six months it is time to see how your child's development and temperament matches the expectations of that particular school and classroom. A "natural mother-killer" may have difficulty with class expectations to sit down, be quiet, and do independent work. You will have made such an assessment before school entry by visiting the school, and perhaps by having a school readiness evaluation done by the school and by your health care provider.

These evaluations are never definitive, so it will not hurt to see how things are progressing. Major developmental advances can happen to a child at this age — especially in a few months.

The main thing is to keep a positive attitude and praise the child's accomplishments. Don't be too worried about letters that are printed "backwards" at kindergarten and first grade. This is very common. It does not necessarily mean a "learning problem."

Many issues may come up at school or at home that might affect how your child is coping with daily life. Use school resources, such as counselors, for your children, and seek help from your health care provider, who will also know of community resources available to help you sort out the issues involved.

This is important if such events have triggered in the child bouts of depression, or anxiety that may manifest itself in over-eating, lethargy, loss of interest in school or a poor self-image. Changing schools tends to disrupt social contacts and may impact academic progress, so attention to how the child is coping with family stresses is important. If left unattended, such patterns might persist and lead to unhealthy and self-destructive habits later.

Several common issues facing families today include moving and parental separation or divorce. Sometimes these happen at the same time. Children are quite resilient, and can cope with many stresses, but they need a kind ear to listen to what may be happening to them from their perspective. This isn't always easy for a parent who is also caught up in an emotional roller-coaster, or even just has many demands on their time.

Take the time you routinely set aside for talking with your child and at least double it during times of family upheavals. Remember, kids will often think they did something to cause a problem between their parents, or that they might be able to fix it.

School Problems

Dr. Phil Nader says: "I routinely ask parents and the child: 'How is school going?' If I get an answer that is the least bit less than 100% enthusiastic, I inquire further about behavior problems, peer relationships and academic progress. A parent can do the same with their child and with the teacher. If a child is not performing well academically, then an assessment of the situation must be made by the teacher and other school personnel as soon as it is detected. Do not let the behavior or learning problem go unchecked to see if it will improve without intervention."

The most common learning problem is a developmental learning problem — which eventually the child will "outgrow." However, unless adjustments and interventions are made, damage will be done, and the child might learn that they "can't learn." This can have long-lasting effects: reform schools and youth detention facilities are full of kids who have or had untreated learning problems.

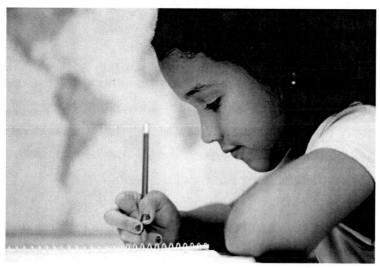

Peer Relationships (Overweight and Other Issues)

At times, kids can be cruel. We can all remember the unfortunate, extremely overweight child in our third grade class, who was teased for her size. We did a study of peer relationships of young school children and found that children who were overweight (over the 85th percentile) were more likely to be "victimized" and feel isolated from their peers. These experiences only cause more isolation and eating for comfort. Being overweight and ridiculed can have other ramifications, such as pushing your child to hang out with other overweight children, where it may be more acceptable to overeat on junk food.

This is a vicious cycle. One must struggle to find sparks of outstanding talent or areas of achievement and ways to reinforce them and recognize them in the overweight child (or any child for that matter.). Sometimes a single friend is all a child needs to repair the damage to her self-concept that such an experience brings. Teachers may also be able to help (e.g., recognition of a socially isolated child's art work or praise for an excellent response in class).

Classroom discussions on differences among people can be helpful in socializing both normal and visibly physically and mentally handicapped children. In life, being able to have a meaningful friendship — even if only one — can go a long way towards a healthy adult adjustment.

Intolerance for differences at this age, avoiding certain gang colors, and differences between well-to-do and

poorer kids, have led many schools to adopt school uniforms.

A recent New Zealand news article which made major headlines there was the finding that school uniforms (which are standard in that country) have greatly expanded to fit the increasing girth of New Zealand schoolchildren! Mediums are now large, and sizes have progressed to XXL!

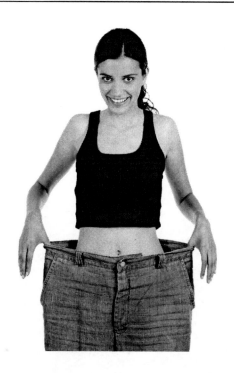

See Chapter 24 for a Summary of Do's and Don'ts: School Age

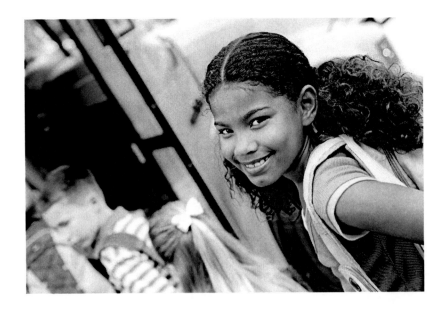

19

MYTH:
Tweens are Unreliable,
and Driven by Fads

Ever heard this? "I'll just DIE if I can't ..."

"But Fran's parents don't care if she (does x, y, z)... !"

"This jacket is too cool!"

"Why can't I (get a tattoo, nose piercing, etc.)?"

REALITY CHECK:

The age period 9–12 years is the time just before adolescence. Tweens are between school age and adolescence. They are at a ripe age to become aware of the discrepancy between what adults say and what they do, and are quick to recognize the hypocrisy — and, of course, feel obligated to criticize those in authority. They can become aware of the manipulation of advertising and media.

One sixth grade class we worked with, during a nutrition series, decided to "take on" the school lunch program. They documented what was being served, calculated calories and fat, and made a presentation to the school board. That resulted in a revision of school food policies, instituting a salad bar option.

Today — all over the country, groups of "tweens" are surveying the food environment, marketing environment and activity opportunities in their neighborhoods, picking priorities and learning to advocate for changes. These programs are instituted by health departments and schools, but there is no reason why a neighborhood association could not also organize their youth to do something similar.

This is an age when the "youngster" starts (literally) to grow up, but they won't reach the start of their adolescent growth spurt until the end of this period around the age of 12 or so; girls generally starting this growth spurt about a year before boys.

While this growing-up period presents challenges to parents, particularly those who can't let go or who feel they need to still baby and control their child, this age is an opportunity for you to spend valuable time enjoying your child, relishing their accomplishments, and reinforcing their feelings of competence and self-confidence, including the wise choices they make about their health. These are the traits that will serve them well in adolescence and young adulthood.

For both boys and girls, a significant growth spurt — rapid increase in height — signals the onset of puberty. Since girls mature earlier, they often become taller in fifth or sixth grade compared to their boy classmates. This may create a powerful social inhibition on being physically active for some girls. Girls may not want to beat the boys in physical challenges, even though they could at this age because of growth differences.

Because the hormones puberty stirs up make it very difficult to "grow into excess weight" (despite the growth spurt), this may be one of your last chances to really keenly monitor the effects of the environment on your child's eating and activity habits, and the packing on of unwanted weight. This is particularly true at the early ages of this period. It is important to know what your child's BMI is as it gives you a sense of how vigilant you need to be in attempting to influence eating and activity habits.

A lot of this influence must be *indirect*.

This is because "prohibiting" certain sedentary activity such as TV watching, or "requiring" healthy food choices like broccoli, are likely to result in resentment and rebellion — either now or later.

So become involved in all aspects of children's lives and experiences at this age. Discuss and debate various topics and issues across the wide range of human existence, such as "world peace."

This fits in very well with the child's expanding range of interests and education, as well as putting you in a good position to be a trusted mentor for later. Know how your child is spending their time, with friends, alone, in shopping malls, at school and at after-school activities. Know your child's friends, their families and neighborhoods.

Watch for opportunities to praise — without making it sound ridiculous — or reinforce those habits and activities that include healthy food choices and physical activity as well as non-smoking and avoiding too-early risk-taking: "Hmm. I can see you really like playing soccer after school. It must be fun."

It isn't unusual to hear of 8 or 9-year-old girls starting dieting, limiting "bad" foods because their friends are thinner or the models in magazines are prettier and thinner. If you encourage your child to continue healthy eating habits and not focusing on the "dieting" behavior, your daughter will eventually come out of the dieting phase and realize (thanks to your support) that she is unique and special the way she is. Encourage those things that make your child unique: "You're a great friend," "I love what a team player you are." **Avoid making any comments whatsoever at this age about "gaining a little weight" or looking heavier or pudgier.**

More Sex Education.

Does your child know the answer to the question of "What is happening to my body?" Tweens must be prepared for what will happen to them!

Just before adolescence begins is a good time to review the sex education facts that you have already provided earlier. It is especially important to have a child knowledgeable about what is going to be happening to his or her body in the next few years — hair growth, increasing size of genitals, wet dreams (how to handle the sheets), menstruation and hygiene. Do not let skin changes, such as pimples and acne, go untreated.

Advanced untreated skin problems can result in physical and emotional scarring. There are many ways to limit the effects, and prevent the progression of early acne: ask your doctor.

You may want to arrange an appointment with their doctor to review their growth and likely changes in their bodies — it is sometimes easier for kids to have this discussion with someone other than you, their parent. Because of modesty at this age, it may be difficult for a parent to be up to date on subtle early body changes such as early pubic or armpit hair. After puberty begins, it isn't unusual for some boys to develop "small breasts"; for those who do, a visit with the doctor can be very reassuring.

Screen Time

Computer games, hand-held games and other new marvels of the electronic age are magnets for this age group. A whole new communication matrix, including text-messaging rather than going down the street to talk with a friend, is evolving.

This holds a possibility for even more reduction of active time, but it need not. You may want to consider "trade outs" from time allotted for TV to allow for recreational cell phone or computer use by your tweenager.

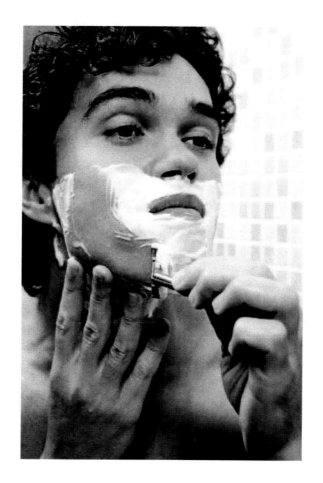

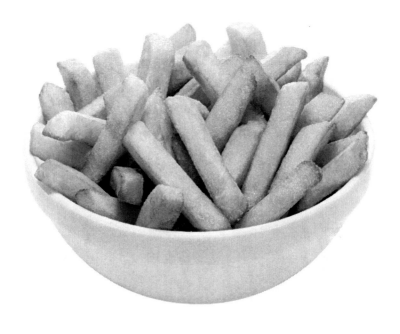

20

MISCONCEPTION:
French Fries Count as a 5-A-Day Vegetable

Ever heard this? "Sure, I ate my vegetables (French
Fries) three times today!"
"What? I can't hear you." (said with
ear phones inserted)
"Just let me get through this
next game"

REALITY CHECK:

Tweens are particularly vulnerable to falling away from the
healthy lifestyle that you have diligently provided at home
over the years! For example, now it is easier just to skip
breakfast, pop in a toaster pastry, and grab and go throughout
the day.

The good news is that while eating and activity are never more chaotic, after this age and the following adolescent period, the earlier patterns tend to be returned to.

Knowing all this, the aware parent can try to maintain and reinforce as many healthy eating routines as are already established in the family. Healthy snack availability after school is never more important than at this age. Interestingly, many parents who have successfully previously instilled healthy preferences report that their pre-teens actually enjoy home-style snacks because of their comfort and familiarity.

Eating Out and On the Run

Often the parent is as caught up in busy schedules as the child, so use the opportunity to make healthy choices when eating out and on the run. Make sure your child sees you making these choices. Again, it is a good idea to do this before adolescence hits with full force.

- Drink water rather than milk shakes or high sugar drinks.
- Have your sandwich without mayo or cheese
- Get dressings (mayo, sauces, sour cream) on the side
- Avoid "all you can eat" places
- Hit the veggies and downplay the fried foods

Fast Food

Instead of ...	*Try ...*
Fried Chicken Sandwich	Grilled chicken sandwich without mayonnaise or cheese
Submarine or deli sandwiches with loads of mayonnaise and cheese and luncheon meats	Turkey meat, loads of veggies, mustard and light mayonnaise
Roast beef sandwich with cheese	Roast beef sandwich with barbecue sauce
Fried chicken and steak tacos	Chicken or steak soft tacos in corn tortillas; skip the guacamole and sour cream
Regular hamburger	Child's hamburger with catsup
Regular hamburger	Grilled veggie burger

McDonald's, as well as other fast food restaurants, have healthy kids' choices, such as cut-up apples instead of fries and 1% milk and water rather than sugary drinks.

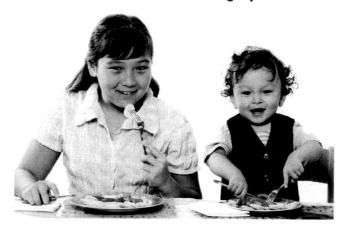

Family Style Restaurants

Instead of...	*Try...*
French fries	Baked potato with sour cream on the side
Croissants or biscuits	Whole-wheat bread, pita pockets or wraps
Cream soups	Broth soups with loads of vegetables
Buttery vegetables	Raw or steamed vegetables
Ice cream	Fruit ice, sherbet, or low-fat yogurt or ice cream

Encouraging Tweens to be Active

Destroy gender and cultural myths! Who says boys can't jump rope, girls can't lift weights, whites can't break dance, boys can't become ballet or tap dancers, and Hispanic girls should not exercise or sweat?

These expectations start gaining a foothold in school age and continue into adolescence. Look for ways to explode these myths and help a child try something they think they would like to do. Kids will generally do what they want to do and are good at, but the activity must fit the child. There are many ways to support activity: do active things as a family;

give praise and encouragement; provide transportation to games, parks, programs, and leagues.

Mostly adults want safety and lack of injury when it comes to sports. This may lead to over-protection. Learn to balance your concerns with allowing your child to give the sport a try if they feel strongly about it. If they fail or are injured, at least they will gain self-confidence by participating.

Organized Sports

At this age, boys and girls are often shunted into gender-specific activities, such as boys' and girls' leagues and teams. Without going into the merits and disadvantages of this separation, there are benefits for participating, especially if the philosophy is just that: participation rather than winning! Try to find out and encourage the activity that your child selects, and can do well, rather than force things that will be difficult (such as tumbling or ballet if the child is large or clumsy). A heavier boy might benefit from activities in which being heavier might be an advantage, such as football or wrestling. A somewhat frail or underweight boy no matter how much he wants to excel, can get hurt playing football. You can judge at this age, and later as they enter adolescence, whether their body matches the sport. Be sure to maintain good communication with adult leaders, coaches and trainers so that you can spot potential trouble spots.

Follow Their Heart!

Remember to allow your child to follow their heart in picking the sport or activity they want, and not what you've always dreamed your child should do. This saves a lot of heartache for both of you. You'll be surprised at the good things that will come your way when a child is happy and supported in their decisions ... better grades, choosing good people to be friends with, self-confidence and so much more.

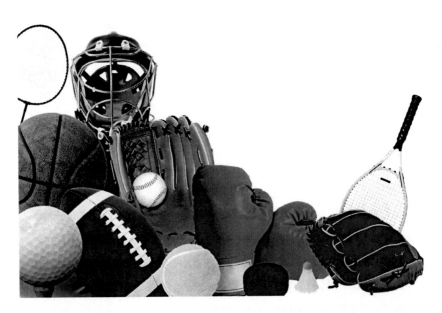

See Chapter 24 for a Summary of Do's and Don'ts for Tweens

21

MYTH:
You Can't Talk with a Teenager

Ever heard this? "Where did you go?" "Out."

"What did you do? "Nothing."

"Why don't you act like an adult?" (They can't — they're not adults.)

REALITY CHECK:

Believe it or not, studies have shown that teens turn most often to their parents and family in times of stress and questioning.

As reassuring as that is, anyone who has raised teens will agree that it is a difficult time because adolescents act like ... well, adolescents! Even though they appear almost "grown up."

Adolescence is also known as "the big hunger." I know you can picture right now a teen — just before and just after dinner — peering into the open refrigerator looking for something to eat!

Tip
Keep plenty — I mean plenty — of healthy snacks available at home!!

- Water

- Cut-up fruit

- Cut-up veggies

- String cheese

- Pretzels

- Non-fat yogurt

- Low or Non-fat milk

This physical hunger also reflects a developmental hunger to solve the three main tasks of adolescence:

- Identity (Who am I?)

- Independence

- Sexuality

The tools they use to wrestle with these issues come from the feelings of trust, confidence, and competence they have gained through the earlier childhood years.

All adolescents will also turn to friends and their peer group both for information and to find out "the thing" to do. Keep up a dialog about almost anything that your teen wants to talk about. Remember, conversation is a two-way street, so this is an age when you can begin to share your everyday thoughts and "battles" — without burdening your teen. Try to model problem solving and how you approach decision-making.

There are many good books on communicating with your teenager, but the easiest way is to *listen* very carefully to see if you can determine any issues that are really important to your teenager and give them a chance to vent — even if you know that their concern is overstated.

There is one topic you should not talk about with your teenager. You really have to back off when it comes to comments about being overweight or fat.

A comment overheard from a middle-aged overweight woman who was jumping rope: "I can still hear my parents telling me how fat I was … and you know what? I did get fat — even though as I look back at pictures of me at the time I really wasn't that fat as a pre-teen" This is an example of how a psychological environment caused over-eating. This over-eating added fat cells during adolescence and resulted in adult obesity.

The opposite of obesity, eating disorders such as anorexia or binge/purge behaviors, may also result from inappropriate comments about the body or appearance. For a while it was thought that the eating/purging behavior was so common among girls that it was just a matter of degree as to whether it became serious enough to be diagnosed and treated. This was a time when the ultra-thin models were prominent in advertising. Fortunately, this is not as emphasized today. Yet one never really sees "ample" models in magazines, TV shows, movies, or ads. Girls get many mixed messages: to be thin and sexy, but also be happy the way they are and have strong morals.

For boys, the usual response is to want to "bulk up" or gain weight. A boy who has anorexia or purges could be suffering from a more severe disorder and needs immediate medical care. If purging and binging is detected in either sex, medical evaluation and intervention is called for.

Research

Adolescents have the cognitive ability to think about something, set it off to the side and analyze it. They can readily see inconsistencies in what parents say and what they do. This is an age when parents become less and less intelligent and knowledgeable and the teen wants to make decisions by themselves. It is only until later that they will appreciate that you might have known a little something!

The answer to "Who am I?" will come in time and not happen overnight; what is true today may not hold for eternity. Spiked, dyed hair may just be a transient view of the look a teen is experimenting with. Deeper identity issues include: who am I — as a friend? buddy? counselor? worker? employee? sibling? future parent? and others.

Career and vocational paths are also set by schooling experiences along the way before and during adolescence. This can play a major role in determining a person's identity. It is not too late to inquire about counseling resources and clubs available in school.

A sudden change in academics may signal some other issues that have come to the forefront, so keep your vigilance up about school, and continue monitoring as best you can what your teen is doing, and who they are hanging out with. Offer your own family room, garage or basement as a social hang-out place or rock band practice site!

Limits and Teenagers

Allowing a teen to gain independence is one of the most challenging tasks for parents. How can this be done without abandoning limits and guidelines for acceptable and non-harmful behavior — to self and to others?

Think of an inverted triangle.

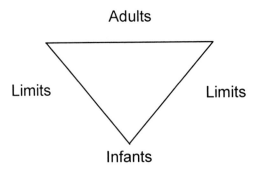

The sides of the triangle represent guidelines or limits. Age increases as you go from the narrowest part to the widest part of the triangle. For infants, almost their entire environment is controlled for their safety and nurturing. Even for adults, there are legal limits for behavior that result in consequences if crossed.

Adolescents are passing through a period when their desire is to cross limits, and parents must learn how to negotiate limits in such a way as to preserve safety as well as nurture independence.

When caught up in this process, it is wise to remember that sometimes it is better to argue over two alternatives — both of which might be acceptable to the parent — just because the teen may want and need the experience of "convincing" you that their position is acceptable, and that they can prove themselves to be "responsible."

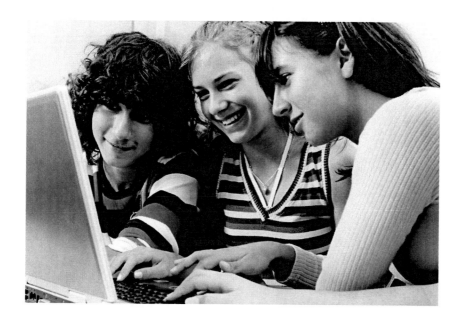

22

MISCONCEPTION:
The Teen Years Are
A Good Time To Try
To Lose Weight

Ever heard this? "Why don't you slim down before the
prom?"
"All you have to do is get up earlier on
Saturday and go for a run."

REALITY CHECK:

Adolescents are much too busy with growing up and the tasks
of adolescence to add on the tough assignment of losing
weight! In fact, it might actually backfire and make weight
loss, if needed, even harder to accomplish.

If your teen already has a few extra pounds or is at a BMI of
85th percentile or higher, you have to wait until they are ready

to decide on their own to attempt to lose weight — which will be as difficult for them as it is for adults to undertake.

There are some instances when teens **are** successful in **losing weight and keeping it off,** but **the key is that the desire comes from within and is not imposed or suggested by others.** The major take-home message is that successful adolescent weight loss programs include a healthy, low-fat diet, plenty of activity, and psychological help to make a permanent change to a healthy lifestyle. Such changes take at least a year to make a significant start, working at it nearly full time. Avoid anything like a fad diet that promises a quick fix!

The main thing to do is to concentrate on things that your teen can do to feel good about themselves, excel in, and make friends. **Do not nag or remind! It only makes the teen feel worse.** And what is the result? You guessed it.

Of course, you will keep up your resolve to have a healthy home environment regarding food and recreation opportunities. Hopefully your teen has already gotten a taste for healthy food and regular exercise; if not, insisting on it now is likely to not be taken well.

Remember, appearance is a major concern in adolescence, so help the teen to dress sharply, be friendly, and find a niche success area. For overweight boys, sometimes participation in weight training and heavy lifting — with a trainer — is ideal.

Girls' activity is influenced tremendously by the peer group and social expectations. If they have already been involved in sports or clubs this can be a trusted source of both activity and friends. The teen years can also become a time when "their choice" of trying something new can result in a positive outcome. Trying tennis for the first time, perhaps partly because the tennis coach is "cute," or cheerleading or marching because of the attention and spotlight that it puts them in still results in activity.

PE and High Schools

A great deal of work needs to be done to improve PE and healthy exercise programs in high schools. This will no doubt require changes in the education codes, as well as a reorientation of the purposes of PE at the high school level. Ideally high school would be the best time for allowing and encouraging life-long activity habits and skills for all students, rather than preparation for JV and varsity sports for only a few.

There should be an "activity period" at the end of the day in which all students — not just the "athletes" — could try out various ways to get an aerobic work out that fits their interests and abilities. Race-walking, dancing, martial arts, and even community service activities with some physical component are possibilities.

The use of high school fields, tracks and gyms on weekends might be a resource that could be supported for teens in a local area.

Providing recreational opportunities for teenagers is important for physical activity. These opportunities also provide a diversion for teenagers who often find themselves pre-occupied with sex at this age. They can't help it, it's the hormones! Sex influences everything. This is also true for adults, but adults are often able to subdue and suppress these influences better than teens who are less experienced and maybe desire more.

Research on Sexual Behavior

Most early sexual behavior is done alone. Masturbation and self-stimulation is normal. Early unprotected intercourse (with either gender) is what most parents fear most — because of the possible consequences of unwanted pregnancy, or acquiring serious diseases. This happens with enough frequency that laws have been passed to permit teens to seek medical care — even without parental permission — to deal with these possible conditions.

Can you establish enough trust and rapport with your teen that you can be available to them in seeking whatever advice or medical help is required to help them mature with responsibility to themselves and others? Arm yourself with knowledge and facts. They will be seeking information from any and all sources, including "street" knowledge and peer information that may be (but more likely isn't) accurate. **Turn to others — a doctor, school counselor — for help if you believe there is a need to communicate with your teen and you or the teenager can't or won't.**

The most desired position for a parent is to have the trust and communication already established so that the teen can approach the parent on any topic. They learn this from previous experience.

If you have given signals that certain topics, such as homosexuality, are taboo, you will not be approached! This could be a tragedy for a confused or questioning teenager concerned about their sexual orientation, or the behaviors of other teens they encounter.

If such a teen feels that they are different or have desires that are unacceptable, it can have a profound effect on their self-image and later ability to function fully as an adult. It may also result in self-destructive behaviors, depression and eating problems, excessive drug use, and even suicide. Would you rather have a gay son or daughter or a dead one?

Beyond Adolescence

There are many more adolescent issues, and they would require more space to deal with than is available in this book. Issues such as smoking, drinking, experimentation with drugs, dating, sexuality, choice of occupation, moral and ethical development, working and dropping out of school, and delinquency, arise in the teenage years and influence health and health habits.

Thankfully, the protective effects of a healthy lifestyle established earlier in life will resurface as "habits" and "desired activities" as the teenage years carry on into young adulthood.

Diet will revert back to healthier choices, and adult "play" — exercise routines and sports — will become an integral part of daily life as a young adult, even though there will be expected deviations from a healthy diet and regular activity because of educational and work demands.

The "obesegenic" environment will not go away easily.

One can always count on the adverse environmental forces encouraging sedentary activity and readily available unhealthy foods to be a factor working against maintaining an optimal weight and being physically fit.

One adolescent-to-adulthood responsibility will be to work for policy and regulatory changes that promote healthy eating and activity in schools, in work sites, and in the general community.

Examples of Policy and Regulatory Efforts

- Access to school grounds for recreational purposes on weekends.

- More required active PE in schools.

- Better access to farmers' markets.

- Control on numbers and density of fast food outlets.

- Traffic policies that make it safer and easier to walk or bike.

See Chapter 24 For A Summary of Do's and Don'ts For Adolescence

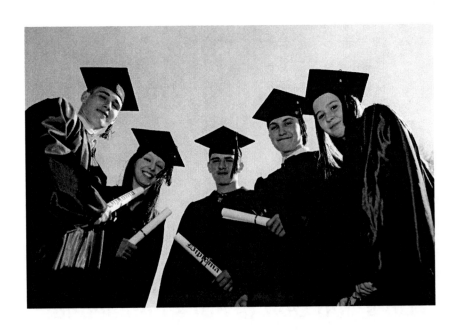

23

From Knowledge To Action

Now that we understand how the *great denial* has prevented us from taking actions that would help us avoid the problem of gaining too much weight, we need to think about what might be keeping us from changing our behavior or the behavior of others, such as businesses, developers, governments, schools, media, chambers of commerce, legislators, the health and fitness industries, farmers and the food industry — that is, all of us!

The easiest but not most obvious step is to stop dwelling on the dangers of being overweight, and keep the knowledge about food and activity you have gained in reading this book "under the radar screen" while you just go about having a fun and enjoyable life. In other words, life itself has so many joys and challenges, preventing obesity should just happen *naturally* because we don't make a big deal out of it.

However, some of us may have to make a big deal out of it, until more of the population is moved to take on the tasks of protecting our kids from the adverse environment out there, and changing the environment so that it naturally supports and encourages our more healthy choices about diet and activity. These choices will then become habits. Eventually the environment will change because everybody agreed it was the "right thing to do."

So, it is really all about **changing behaviors and habits.**

Steps in Behavior Change - Where are you?

- Not even thinking about it.
- Becoming aware that a change might be a good thing.
- Thinking about making a change.
- Understanding your current behavior, what triggers it, what keeps it going.
- Setting goals and making a plan to change — change should be in small, doable steps.
- Carrying out the plan.
- Checking on how the plan worked, and modifying it.
- Preparing for setbacks and relapses into old habits.
- Looking for support to turn the change into a habit.

We hope that after reading this book, you will find yourself on this spectrum of behavior change and use it to mark your progress in establishing a healthier lifestyle for yourself and your kids. (Refer to the worksheet in the next chapter on setting behavioral goals.)

Below are *ten ways* that parents or parents-to-be can protect their child against obesity every day:

1. Be informed.

- Know all you can about food and fitness.

- Know all about the child you get. Every child is different.

- Know what you are up against in your environment.

2. Be a skilled provider.

- Make good choices for your family.

3. Be a good detective of the environment.

- Identify and resist bad influences.

- Identify and reinforce good influences.

4. Negotiate support.

- Involve family and friends.

5. Deal with opposition.

- Expect complaints.

- Stay calm.

6. No nagging; have fun.

- Know when to lighten up.

- Emphasize having fun.

7. Read labels.

- Focus on the fine print.

- Know your foods from the inside out.

8. Activate!

- Match the activity to the kid.

- Advocate for parks, and school and community policies promoting health.

9. Tell others.

- Share your ideas and knowledge.

10. Trust you have done the best you can.

- Have faith in yourself and your child.

In addition to being a parent (and even if you are not a parent), you can engage where you might be able to make some changes — no matter how small — in factors that impact the environment today.

Pediatrician and Family Physician — make obesity prevention a priority by counseling and activating parents with sound child development principles, limiting screen time, monitoring children's growth, and building a local community referral resource for families to learn about nutrition and engage in activity. Be an active advocate for good preschool and school nutrition and PE programs.

OB-GYN — monitor healthy weight goals during pregnancy, and promote breastfeeding.

Health Care Payers and Insurers — provide for evaluation and long-term cost benefit analysis of prevention efforts, and pay for implementation of effective prevention activities.

Businessperson — set up work site wellness and health programs for employees, provide facilities for breastfeeding mothers, and request health plans to reward enrollees for fitness efforts for themselves and for their kids. Advocate for healthy schools and communities to attract a healthy workforce.

Legislator — introduce and pass legislation regarding healthy snacks and drinks in public places like schools and government agencies, and consider legislation controlling numbers of fast food outlets and accessibility of fresh fruits and vegetables. Investigate the role of government subsidies for foods that are the staple ingredients of fast and processed foods. Watch for growing inequity of healthy environments in less affluent communities.

Local Government — review policies and procedures that can be modified to increase opportunities for activity and healthy nutrition, and require health impact statements for new development and redevelopment projects.

Advertising — produce pro-bono or public awareness messages on prevention of obesity to counter the huge amount of advertising of unhealthy products and services.

Food industry — market healthy food items, portions and choices at reasonable prices. Through advertising, set consumer preferences for more healthy foods.

Faith-Based — be aware of types of food and activity offered to parishioners at social and fellowship dinners and fund-raisers. Have a responsibility to make members aware of the relationship between a healthy diet and weight management, and of particular risks that the congregation may have due to their race or ethnicity, such as hypertension or diabetes.

Media — feature stories and series that highlight efforts and research dealing with obesity prevention. Cease advertising to young children.

Planning and Development — make arrangements for increased use of parks and recreational spaces, bike and walking paths, and playgrounds.

Transportation — work to improve accessibility and walkability, and traffic control.

Educator — consider health first when dealing with preschool and school policies regarding PE and nutrition, recess, school foods and snacks, parties, and club fund-raising.

WIC Worker — promote parent education on nutrition and healthy shopping, and monitor children's growth.

Remember all these policy-level and societal changes need ordinary individuals to become informed and work with policymakers to place priorities where they should be!

How Does Society Make Such Changes?

This should not take the thirty years it has taken to get us where we are. Recall how seat belt use and infant car seats were viewed as an infringement on personal liberties that undermined mother–infant bonding? In less than a decade, a new idea that was embraced by more and more people became a social norm. The same thing can happen with preventing obesity.

The United States just fell to 43rd in ranking for life expectancy among countries of the world, a lower ranking than some developing countries. The culprits: obesity and lack of health care. These are potentially powerful motivators for change in our society. But a two-tiered approach is required: grass roots awareness with personal and collective action, paired with a governmental willingness to examine policy and regulations.

The barriers to action, beyond the values and beliefs that impinge on this problem, are the classic ones: time and money.

It is clear where most money is spent and earned: in ways that promote an unhealthy lifestyle. There have been many parallels drawn between smoking and the obesity epidemic, in terms of promotion, taxation, and ill effects. To date, there is promising hope from several philanthropies and foundations such as the Robert Wood Johnson Foundation, the California Endowment and others, to help communities engage at both the grass roots and policy levels. There is no clear source, at present, of a universal approach to funding obesity prevention efforts. Part of this is because there are so many sectors of society that affect the issue.

Time is always a constraint. So here are some things you can do with varying amounts of time.

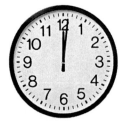

If you have 1 minute:

- Catch your child doing something healthy and praise them. "Way to go kicking that soccer ball around." "I love the way you're snacking on baby carrots."

- Wash a bunch of grapes or apples and set them in the refrigerator where all can see and have access to them.

- Pour cold water into a sports bottle for you and your child to drink throughout the day.

- Discuss your child's favorite activities. Favorite fruits and veggies?

- Cut your restaurant meal in half and put the rest in a doggie bag for later.

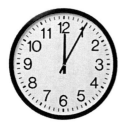

If you have 5 minutes:

- Cut up an apple for you and your child.

- Fill celery sticks with peanut butter and sprinkle with raisins.

- Put baby carrots on a plate with low-fat ranch dressing.

- Wash all fruit and put in a bowl in the refrigerator.

- Show your children how to do some simple stretches. Breathe.

- Set the timer for 5 minutes and have your children run around the house, helping to pick up.

- Post a healthy eating and/or a physical activity goal on the refrigerator. Involve your family in deciding what these goals should be, and what kinds of healthy rewards will be given once they are achieved.

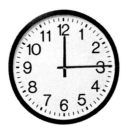

If you have 15 minutes:

- Walk with your family around the neighborhood.

- Grate veggies and put them into whatever meal you're making for the evening meal, such as soup, quesadillas, casseroles, etc.

- Go outside and kick a ball around with your child.

- Walk the dog.

- Make a fruit smoothie with fresh fruit, non-fat yogurt, ice, juice.

- Help your child make their lunch for school. Write an encouraging note on their napkin.

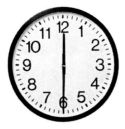

If you have 30 minutes:

- Walk with your family for 30 minutes. Let your children pick the route.

- Find a recipe with your child that contains loads of

vegetables. Make a grocery list with the items needed to prepare the recipe. If you include your child in either the shopping or the preparation of the meal — they're more likely to try new foods.

- Make a grocery list with all the healthy items you and your family need for the week. Research has shown that 60–70% of what ends up in your cart is unplanned. So plan ahead and shop the periphery of the store where you'll find the majority of the healthy items. A healthy grocery list is included in the next chapter.

- Do an activity with your family that you've never done. Have your child choose the activity.

- Pretend you're a kid for 30 minutes. Go outside and run around with your children like you used to do when you were a child.

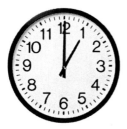

If you have 1 hour:

- Take your children grocery shopping with you. Remember your list. Have them pick out the apples. Have them choose their favorite low-fat or non-fat yogurt.

- While your child is at soccer or dance practice for an hour, get the other mothers and fathers around you to go for a walk instead of sitting around waiting.

- Plan a week's menu.

- Go to a park. Play on the monkey bars, slide down the slides with your children.

- Make dinner instead of ordering out or going out to dinner.

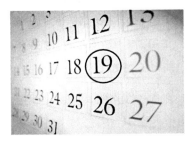

If you have 1 day:

- Visit the school or day care center your child attends.

- See what activity and eating arrangements are practiced.

- Organize parents to advocate for daily activity and healthy food.

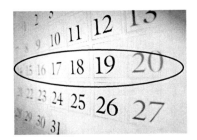

If you have 1 week or longer:

- Organize neighborhood parents to lobby the school to change the recess and PE policies.

- Visit with elected officials to advocate for greater accessibility of recreation facilities.

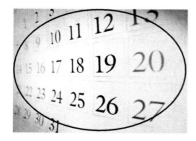

If you have 1 month or longer:

- Embark on a personal makeover that focuses on healthy living habits, and enjoyable activity. Weight loss and body toning will happen naturally.

- Organize a community vegetable garden.

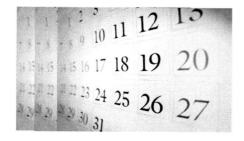

If you have 1 to 5 years or more:

- Engage with others to forge multi-sector partnerships to attack the problem of obesity at a community wide level. It is amazing what can be done collectively by busy people who share a common value of fighting the problem of obesity in kids. Set doable goals, try to base efforts on data, and measure the impact on people, programs, institutions and communities. Do what you can to raise awareness in the general public and in targeted specific interest groups.

- Value diversity and the role of cultures and traditions in addressing obesity prevention. Use both a tree-top and a grass roots approach. Make sure they are connected to each other. Multiply your effectiveness by engaging volunteer partners in all sectors of society. Be open and transparent, and value the contributions of others.

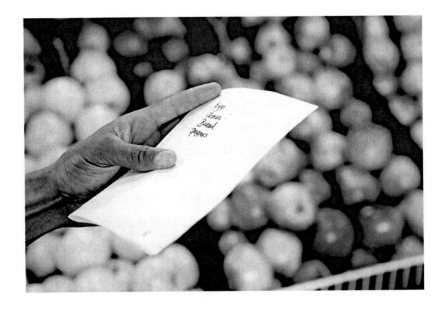

24

Rules and Tools
To Protect
Kids From Obesity

These new rules are based upon the principles of child development and the findings of the latest research in nutrition and physical activity. They are discussed in more detail in previous sections in the book, corresponding to these ages and stages of development.

After the rules are some tools and worksheets you will find helpful in watching the "in" side of the energy equation; some helpful shopping and food preparation tactics; how to calculate and interpret your child's body mass index; and how to set a health goal and achieve it.

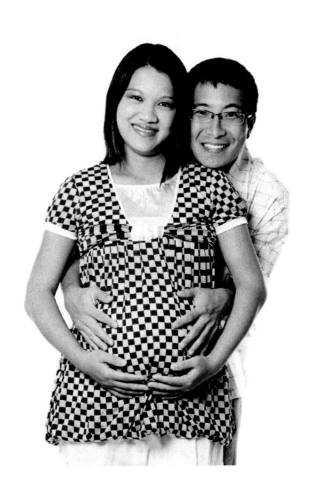

Pregnancy

DO

- Have cut-up fruit in the refrigerator. Wash and drain spinach leaves for an easy-to-make salad. Have almonds and whole-grain bread in your cupboard. **You're more likely to eat better, and later your children will too, if your home is set up to make eating healthy easy.**

- The amount of recommended weight gain depends upon your initial body mass index or BMI. For the average weight woman (BMI 19.8–26.0), about one pound per week during the 2nd and 3rd trimesters — or a total of about 25–35 pounds is suggested. If carrying twins, slightly larger weight gain is expected.

- Drink at least 32 ounces of water.

- Fill up on fiber by eating whole-grain breads and cereals, as well as dried beans, legumes and nuts.

- Eat every 3 to 4 hours. This will maintain your blood sugar level, you'll have more energy throughout the day, and you'll be less likely to binge.

- Eat sweets and fats every once in a while. You've seen what happens when you try to deny yourself that candy bar — you end up eating three instead of the one you wanted in the first place. Treat yourself to low-fat frozen yogurt instead of ice cream. Instead of eating the entire candy bar, eat half of it. Choose baked chips instead of regular chips.

DO

- Get early and regular prenatal health care. In addition to taking good care of yourself during pregnancy, this is a period when you have a little time to consider what things you want to emphasize when you have your own children, in order for them to grow up as healthy as they can. This can include decisions about breastfeeding, getting immunizations and general child rearing.

- Walking during and after pregnancy is a great way to limit the effects of eating "for two," and will also counter the tendency to cut down on your normal active lifestyle during and after pregnancy.

DON'T

- Neglect your healthy lifestyle and other habits. Routine daily exercise, adequate sleep, stress-avoidance and parenting education are all helpful when considering pregnancy. If you smoke, you will never find a more important time or reason to quit.

- Avoid sex if you feel like it. Check with your OB if you have any questions.

- Use drugs and alcohol if you are pregnant, or are planning pregnancy. The investment you put into your own health and well-being will pay dividends not only to you, but also to your child.

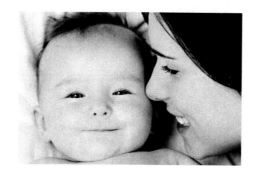

Infancy

DO

- Breastfeed exclusively for the first 6 months. Get help and support to feed breast milk even if you have to return to work. At the start, feed every 2-3 hours for 10 minutes each breast.

- Prepare fresh first foods at home rather than using store-bought processed baby foods with added, unneeded sugar. It's cheaper too.

- Learn how to interpret weight and height growth charts for your baby. Watch for signs of normal growth. Look for rapid increases in weight compared to length. After age 2, learn how to calculate your child's BMI (body mass index).

- Start to observe your child's personality (from at least 3 months onward). Every child is different and will react in different ways to new foods, situations and general mood. You will have to learn to know the child you get. If you do, it will help with raising them the way you want to.

- Think about the way you were raised. Are there things you want to continue or change for your own child?

DON'T

- Fall into the trap of thinking that a fat baby is necessarily a healthy baby.

- Top-off breast feeds with a bottle, or later put a young child to bed with a bottle "for comfort" If bottle-feeding, 32 ounces per day is recommended.

- Panic about crying up to 2–3 hours a day (usually around 6 weeks of age). This is normal "exercise"; if baby is recently fed, with diapers changed, he or she does not require additional feeding.

- Punish any infant or child between birth and 2 years.

- Get upset if food is played with — everything is played with at this age, smeared around and dropped on the floor!

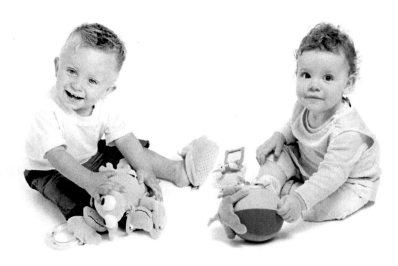

Preschool Age (2 to 4½ Years)

DO

- Give two choices rather than say "no."

- Distract and redirect rather than oppose a 2-year-old.

- Use healthy foods and snacks, but only child-size portions. If your child leaves food on the plate, put less food on the plate next meal.

- Use low-fat or skim milk after age 2.

- Serve small portions, avoid the "Clean Plate Club."

- Encourage active play outside at least 1 hour a day.

- Limit TV to 1–2 hours per day.

- Investigate day care settings regarding nutrition and activity.

DON'T

- Worry about a decreased appetite from 2–4 years — it's normal. One real meal a day is common.

- Say, "Ah, come on, honey, just one more bite," or "You can have some candy if you finish your plate."

- Have a "candy stash" drawer, or prolong Halloween or Easter candy more than one day.

- Constantly tell children to "stop running around," "be careful," "slow down," or "sit down and watch TV."

DON'T

- Add a TV to a child's bedroom.

- Put the child down when correcting him: "You are bad," instead of "What you did was bad."

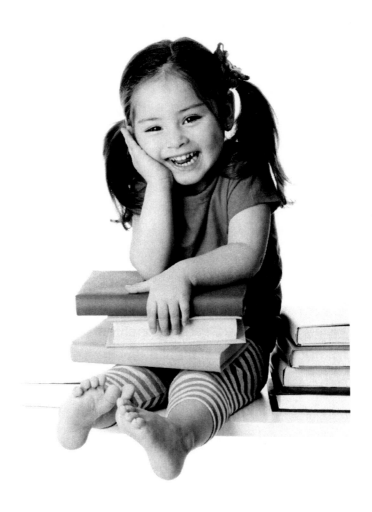

School Age (5 to 9 Years)

DO

- Check your child's BMI at 5–7 years.

- Remember, per day:

    - 5 servings of fruits or vegetables

    - 4 glasses of water (replacing some of the soda)

    - 3 servings of low-fat dairy or meat

    - 2 hours of screen time

    - 1 hour (at least) of physical activity (Courtesy CLOCC)

- Show healthy food choices by example.

- Know how your child is doing with:

    - Learning

    - Family and friends

    - Sexual development information.

- Have expected chores and responsibilities for kids.

DON'T

- Go overboard with fats and sugar during celebrations (but do celebrate).

- Assume everything is OK at school... ask your child and the teacher.

- Wait until adolescence to talk with your child about where babies come from (and tell the truth!).

DON'T

- Assume that all food at school is healthy or that kids have daily opportunities to be active.

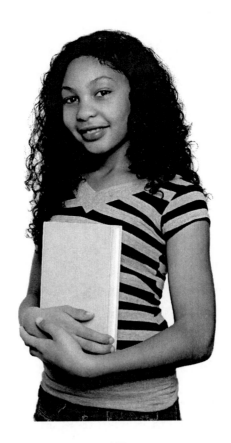

Tweens (9 to 12 Years)

DO

- Prepare you child for puberty and the changes to their body.

- Know who your child's friends are.

- Allow your child to follow their heart regarding activity.

- Engage in as much dialog on all topics as possible.

- Show your child how to choose healthy options at fast food and corner stores.

DON'T

- Discount your child's capacity to become a force, with others, for changes in school and neighborhood policies to improve the activity and nutrition environment.

- Try to parent using force or dictatorial styles.

- Try to parent with no limits whatsoever!

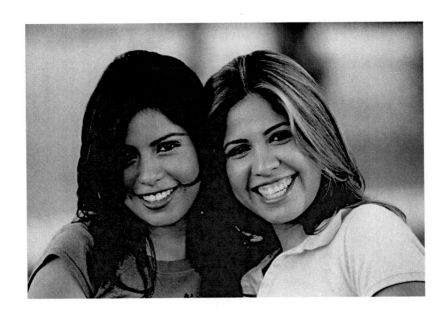

Adolescence (12 Years Plus)

DO

- Have **plenty** of healthy snacks available:

  - Water

  - Cut-up fruit

  - Cut-up vegetables

  - String cheese

  - Pretzels

  - Non-fat yogurt.

- Know the **three tasks** of adolescence

  - Identity (Who am I?)

  - Independence

  - Sexuality

- Keep communication going with your teen (read a book on talking with a teenager).

- Discuss how you go about solving problems and making decisions.

- Inquire at school about school progress and career or college counseling opportunities.

DON'T

- Talk with an overweight (or any) teen about losing weight.

- Refuse to deal with any hint of an issue your teen might have with experimentation in the areas of drugs, smoking, sex, dating or friends.

- Forget to praise and reinforce all those great things that your teenager does.

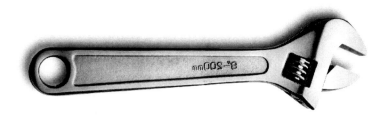

Tools You Need To Balance The "In" Side Of The Energy Equation

Below are examples of amounts of the various food groups for preschoolers and school age kids, based upon the **food pyramid.**

Preschoolers (ages 2–5) and Children (ages 6–11)

Note: daily amounts are given in ranges. If your child is closer to 5, or more active, then use the higher end. If younger or less active, stay on the lower end.

Fruits

Fresh, frozen, canned (in light syrup or water) or dried fruit are all good choices. Fruit juices count, but use occasionally. They are full of calories, and don't have all the nutrients of their fresh counterparts.

Recommended amount per day for **preschoolers**: 1–1½ cups

Recommended amount per day for **children**: 1½ cups

One cup =
> 1 small apple or ½ large apple
> 1 large banana
> 8 large strawberries
> 1 cup of fruit pieces
> 1 cup of 100% fruit juice
> ½ cup of dried fruit

Vegetables

Choose a variety of vegetables. Think the rainbow. You can have purple cabbage, red tomatoes, pumpkins, yellow squash and cauliflower. The deeper and richer the color, the better the vegetable is for you. Fresh, and frozen are best, but canned (if rinsed to get rid of the sodium) are also good choices. Beans and peas can count toward the daily allowance for vegetables.

Recommended amount per day for **preschoolers**: 1–1½ cups

Recommended amount per day for **children**: 2½ cups

One cup =

>1 cup of raw or cooked vegetable pieces
>
>1 cup of vegetable juice
>
>2 cups of leafy vegetables, such as spinach
>
>1 cup of cooked beans, such as pinto beans, black beans, kidney beans
>
>2 medium carrots
>
>1 large tomato

Grains

At least half of the grains eaten should be whole, such as oatmeal, 100% whole-wheat bread, brown rice or wheat pasta.

Recommended amount per day for **preschoolers**: 3–5 ounces

Recommended amount per day for **children**: 6 ounces

1 ounce =

>1 cup ready-to-eat cereal
>
>½ cup of cooked pasta, rice, or cooked cereal
>
>1 slice of bread
>
>¼ bagel from a bagel store
>
>5 whole-wheat crackers
>
>7 square or round crackers
>
>1 pancake
>
>1 tortilla (corn or small whole-wheat flour)

Meat and Beans

Choose lean meats, such as white-meat chicken or turkey, fish, lean or extra-lean beef, pork and other meats. Eat meat alternatives, such as beans, peas, nuts and seeds. These are high in protein; beans and peas are naturally low in fat; nuts and seeds contain good fat; and all are high in protein.
Recommended amount per day for **preschoolers**: 2–4 ounces

Recommended amount per day for **older children**: 5 ounces

1 ounce =
        1 ounce of lean meat, poultry, or fish
        1 regular slice of sandwich meat
        1 egg
        1 tablespoon peanut butter
        ¼ cup cooked beans
        ½ ounce nuts or seeds
        ¼ cup tofu

Milk

Many people are allergic to milk and dairy products, and thrive without it. No adult animals drink milk. When they are thirsty, they drink water. There are bountiful calories in milk, even low fat variety. When choosing milk products choose the low –fat or non-fat items.

Recommended amount per day for **preschoolers**: 2 cups

Recommended amount per day for **older children**: 3 cups

One cup =
> 1 cup of low-fat (1%) or skim (non-fat) milk
> 1 8-ounce container of yogurt
> 1½ cups natural cheese, such as cheddar and Jack cheeses
> 1/3 cup of shredded cheese
> 1½ cups of low-fat ice cream, ice milk or frozen yogurt

Oils

Oils are not a food group per se, but you need some for good health. Choose oils such as olive, canola, and soybean when cooking or choosing a salad dressing.

Other things to keep in mind:

Know how to limit fats and sugars.

- Get your fat and sugar facts on the label.
- Limit solid fats. These are the fats that are solid at room temperature, including butter, margarine, shortening, etc. Limiting these kinds of fat includes limiting the foods that are made with them.
- Choose foods and beverages low in or without added caloric sweeteners, such as fructose, corn syrup, honey and sugars.

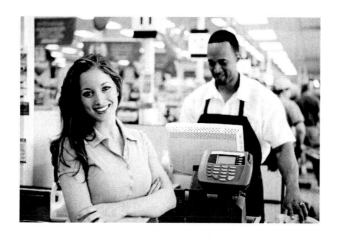

Grocery Store Shopping Tips

Here are some shopping tips that will help you avoid pushing the calories up.

Before Shopping

- Never go to the grocery store hungry. You will buy more than you need, and probably all the comfort foods that are usually high in fat and calories, like cookies and chips.

- Bringing your children is an excellent idea, especially if they are old enough to *not* be influenced by the TV advertising and eye-level placement of candy they will encounter. Remember, they're more likely to eat the fruit or veggies they help pick out than if they weren't considered in the decision. However, be sure you have specific items you "need" their help with or you're going to be held hostage in the cereal and candy aisles.

- Make a shopping list (see next Tool). Think about the meals and ingredients you'll need to purchase. Going without a list means trouble. Not only do you end up buying extra food (and calories) you don't need, but you won't have anywhere to store it ... except on your hips.

While At The Store

- Shop the perimeter of the store where the healthiest foods, including dairy and fresh produce, are found. The unhealthy items are in the middle aisles — try to avoid them if possible.

- Choose **fresh fruits and veggies** that are firm, ripe and unblemished. Purchase only what you can store and eat over the next few days to avoid throwing a whole bunch of produce away. Try to eat at least five servings of fruits and vegetables per day. Tip: Choose tomatoes, which are good for your heart, and red and blue berries, which are loaded with vitamins, minerals and phytochemicals (cancer-fighting chemicals).

- Choose frozen fruits and vegetables if you can't find fresh produce or if you have to store the produce longer than fresh will last.

Eat whole fresh fruits instead of drinking fruit juice or eating dried fruit. These last two ways of getting your fruit are higher in calories and don't have as many vitamins and minerals as their fresh counterpart.

- Try to get your family turned onto *fish*, which contain healthy oils for your heart.

- Choose smart protein. That is, meats that are low in fat like **skinless chicken and turkey breast (white) meat or extra lean ground beef.** Even better, try **legumes and beans**, such as pinto, black and garbanzo beans, and lentils, which are low in fat, and high in protein and fiber. Nuts, especially almonds, are excellent sources of good oils. But watch out — they are also high in calories. An average serving of almonds is six nuts.

- Choose **100% whole-grains**, oats and fibrous foods. Stay clear of white, processed breads and baked goods. Fiber fills you up and creates a healthy digestive tract.

- Cook with **unsaturated fats,** such as olive, canola, and soybean oils. These are considered good for your heart. Watch the amount of oil you use. All oils are chock-full of calories.

- Select **low-fat (1%) or non-fat dairy** products. These foods are high in calcium and protein, and may help in enhancing weight loss.

- Switch to water, if you haven't already. Drinking soda is directly related to weight gain.

- **Read labels.** The smaller the number of ingredients in a prepared product, the healthier. If you don't recognize some of the ingredients listed, then find a product you do understand.

Tip

Don't have time to wash and cut up fruits and veggies? Buy ready-to-eat produce. It's guaranteed to be eaten (instead of throwing away the spinach bunch that never got used). It may be more money up front, but you'll save money in the long run.

Once at home:

- Wash fruit and put in a bowl in the refrigerator.

- Cut up celery and carrots for a quick, healthy snack.

- Chill water.

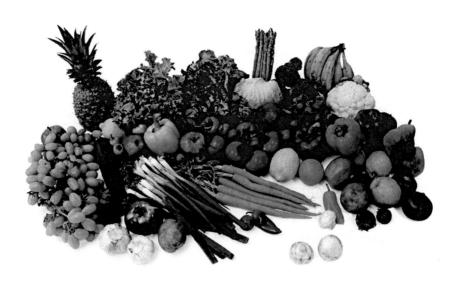

Healthy Grocery List

Take this handy healthy grocery list to help you shop!

Fresh Vegetables

Lettuce	Other greens	Cucumbers	Carrots
Asparagus	Zucchini	Radishes	Tomatoes
Green beans	Onions	Green onions	Peppers
Cauliflower	Broccoli	Peas	Celery
Potatoes	Corn	Sweet potatoes	Squash

Fresh Fruits

Bananas	Apples	Oranges	Pears
Peaches	Nectarines	Grapefruit	Berries

Frozen Foods

Green beans	Peas	Mixed vegetables	Carrots
Chicken breasts	Fruit juice bars	Blueberries	Corn
Fish fillets	Onions	Vegetarian burgers	Shrimp

Canned Foods

Black beans	Tomatoes	Marinara sauce	Tuna
Salmon	Pinto beans	White beans	Pineapples

Meats

Lean hamburger	Pork chops	Steaks	Fish
Shellfish	Chicken	Turkey	Ham

Grains and cereals

Whole-grain bread	Whole-grain pasta	Whole-grain cereal	Oatmeal

Beverages

100% fruit juice	Sparkling water	Tomato juice	Herb tea

Dairy and Eggs

Low-fat sour cream	Low-fat 1% milk	Cheddar cheese	Butter
Low-fat cream cheese	Colby cheese	Mozzarella cheese	Yogurt
Non-fat dairy			

Miscellaneous

Herbs and spices	Sesame oil	Low-fat dressings	Mustard
Low-fat mayonnaise	Honey	Low sodium soy sauce	Walnuts
Pumpkin seeds	Mixed nuts	Almonds	Pecans
Flax seeds	Olive oil	Walnut oil	Garlic

Source http://nutrition.about.com/library/bl_grocery.htm

Setting Health Goals and Achieving Them

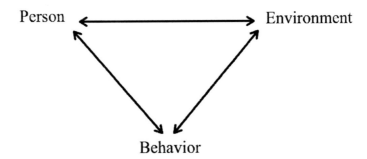

This little diagram does a good job showing one of the major theories of what influences people's behaviors related to their health, such as eating and activity behaviors. It is called Social Learning Theory, and was developed by Albert Bandura from Stanford University. We have used it in many research projects to understand health behavior change, and to assist people to adopt or change a health behavior.

It shows the influence on each other of three crucial elements to consider when attempting to change or adopt a new health behavior. The person actively affects the behavior and is affected by the environment, and each one affects the others. Unless you deal with all three, attempts to change behavior will likely fail.

This is why you cannot just tell people to change health habits, people must be engaged in the process. It is also the rationale for changing the environment (more outdoor play space and healthy snacks) in order to increase children's activity and healthy eating.

Action Plan

The Goal	
How to reach the goal	
Who will be involved?	
When will I/we start?	
What resources will I/we need to make it happen?	
How can I get support (if needed) from: • Friends • Family • Work	
How will I/we know my/our progress towards the goal?	
Date goal reached:	

This will help you fill out the action plan:

Selecting the goal. The goal should be something you are really motivated to do. Ask yourself: why do I really want to do this? Your goal should be less than what you want to eventually do. For example, if you want to run a mile three times per week, and you are currently not even doing brisk walking once a week, brisk walking would be the place to start. Make the goal as specific as you can: "Briskly walk for 30 minutes once per week on Sunday."

How to reach the goal. What will you or others have to do in order to make it happen? Think of things that keep you from doing the goal right now: is it time, equipment, safety, other responsibilities or weather? You may find that several strategies are required to result in a single act of walking 30 minutes once a week on Sunday.

Who will be involved? Think about those who are likely to be able to support you in this effort, and those who might need to change their expectations of you in order for this to happen. Be sure to tell someone about your intentions to carry out your goal. Once you have stated your intention out loud to someone else, you are more likely to succeed!

When will I /we start? It is good to set a specific time and date to begin your goal, not just "soon."

What resources are needed? This means both physical resources (e.g. a place, good walking shoes, comfortable clothes, rain gear if needed, and directions or maps) and encouragement from significant others, maybe even a walking "partner" who also wants to do more activity.

How can I get support?

Social support is one of the determinants of accomplishing your goals. If a family goal is set, each member of the family can devise a way to support another family member to help reach the goal. If your goal is to be able to use a breast pump at work in order to continue feeding your infant breast milk, you will need support from employers and co-workers.

How will I/we assess progress? Keep a written record of what exactly you do. If you don't walk, what were the barriers? Use this information not to feel bad, but to come up with new strategies you may need to employ. Give yourself time to reach your goal, and allow for backsliding. If your goal is too difficult to achieve, it could be too ambitious, and you may need to revise it.

Date goal reached. This is generally a good time to congratulate yourself, and give yourself a reward that is likely to reinforce your aim, e.g. a new warm sweater to wear when it gets cooler during your walks. It also may signal a time to set another more ambitious goal, e.g. walking 3 times a week: twice during the week, once on Sunday.

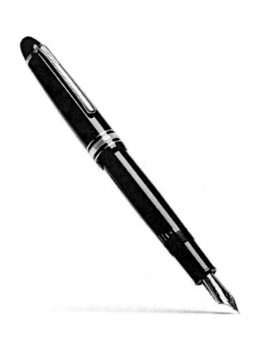

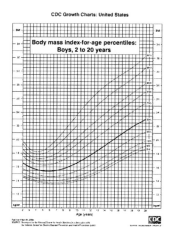

Body mass index-for-age percentiles:
Boys, 2 to 20 years

How To Calculate and Interpret Your Child's BMI (Body Mass Index)

When to use BMI. You can calculate your own or your child's BMI at any time after age 2 years. Without dwelling on it, you might want to check it annually to see the pattern of growth of BMI.

How to calculate it. There is a very easy way to get the BMI number. On the internet, go to: http://cdc.gov/nccdphp/dnpa/ bmi. This will open a page that gives you a choice between an adult BMI calculator and a child/teen BMI calculator. This page also has links on it to tell you more about BMI. Follow the directions and enter the birth date, date of measurement, the height and weight and gender (boy or girl), then click "calculate" and the site will display the number along with the BMI percentile. If you wish you can enter the number on the BMI charts provided in this book.

How to interpret the BMI

A trend — several annual or semi-annual determinations — is better than a single measurement, but if you have old records of heights and weights at different ages you can get a sense of the path of your child's BMI. Many expert groups have defined the following categories:

Under Weight	Less than 5th percentile
Normal Weight	Between 5th and 85th percentile
Over Weight	Between 85th and 95th percentile
Obese	95th percentile and over

It is possible for very muscular teenagers to have a high BMI because they have large muscle mass, but for the most part a high BMI indicates increased body fat.

The above categories are arbitrary. You need to know that the risk of becoming overweight later in life increases the higher your BMI is over the 50th percentile.

What to do if your child's BMI approaches the "overweight" and "obese" categories. The first thing to do is to be a nutrition and activity detective:

- What is the intake of fresh fruits and vegetables?
- How much outdoor play is there?
- Are there safe places to bike, skip rope, and be active at least an hour a day?

- How much time is spent in sedentary activities such as computer games and TV?

- How often and what quality is PE in the school?

Tend to the basic opportunities, make sure they are in place, then follow along for a 6–12 months to see the progress of "growing into" the weight. Your doctor can help with this process. Remember 5, 4, 3, 2, 1

5 fruits and vegetable servings a day
4 glasses of water a day
3 servings of low-fat meat or dairy
2 hours of TV or screen time per day
1 hour or more of active play per day

(Courtesy of the Consortium to Lower Obesity in Chicago Children — CLOCC)

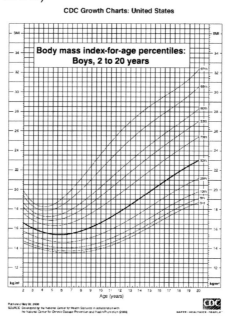

CDC Growth Charts: United States

Body mass index-for-age percentiles: Boys, 2 to 20 years

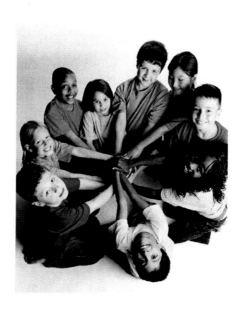

Dealing with Ethnic and Cultural Foods

There are several important issues in relation to regional, ethnic, and cultural differences that seem at first glance to be at odds with healthy nutrition.

ISSUE #1.

What is the meaning of the food dishes or manner of food preparation?

- Family favorite foods usually have a tradition of being passed down through the generations, they may have religious significance, or simply be the wonderful taste of Grandmother's Ribs and Potato Salad. Many times these recipes have been written down.

- Use healthy modern ingredients (such as vegetable oils rather than lard or bacon drippings — or cut down the amounts of "hard" fats).

- Use half the amounts of fatty elements and sugar — likely not to influence the taste that much.

- Use the original recipe but cut the portion sizes.

- Compensate for the extra caloric load on this special occasion by increasing activity.

ISSUE #2.

Know what the real tradition is.

- For example, the traditional native Mexican diet has many fresh fruits, vegetables and fish in it, with corn flour tortillas. Only more recently have refried beans replaced black beans and rice, and white flour replaced corn tortillas.

ISSUE #3.

Use your nutrition knowledge to:

- Evaluate the content of recipes you are trying to make in a healthier way.

- Look especially for sources of calories — sugar and fats.

- If you or your family members just can't stand the taste of the modified version, serve smaller portions of the original recipe on smaller plates.

- Compensate for an occasional splurge with more activity.

ISSUE #4.

Honor the tradition.

- These traditions are important to people and families. They have become important social connections and rituals that relate to a strong family and social sense of well-being. This element is important to maintain — there is much more to eating food together than just the type or kind of ingredients contained in that food. You can alter the content without sacrificing the tradition.

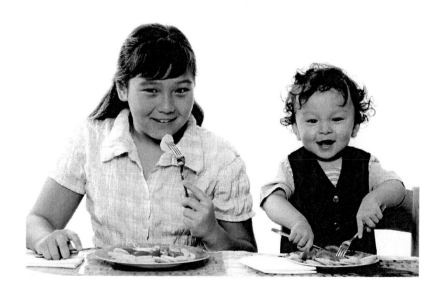

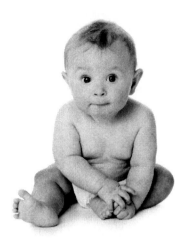

Acknowledgements

Many people contributed directly or indirectly to the ideas and format of this book. The information contained in it is not particularly wild or speculative; much of it is reasoned commonsense based upon scientific research that is out there for anybody to access. We want to get your own reactions and ideas about the topics and usefulness of this book, and welcome your input to the authors.

Email us at pnader@ucsd.edu and mzive@ucsd.edu or at our website **www.youcanpreventchildhoodobesity.org**.

Special thanks are in order to Katherine Kaufer Christoffel M.D., Kristen Copeland, M.D., Suzanne Dixon, M.D., Tim Haft, C.P.T., Fran Kaufmann, M.D., Gene Nathan, M.D., Laura Nathansen M.D., Heather Nichols, M.D., Marion Obrien, Ph.D, Tom Robinson, M.D., Ed Schor, M.D.,Martin Stein, M.D., and Philip D. Szold, M.D., who shared their pediatric, child development and medical expertise in reviewing concepts in the book.

Friends and contacts in the writing and publishing field: Adam Chromy, Peter Janssen and Glenn Vecchione who shared their ideas and suggestions. Thanks also to Alison Southby for editing, Gary Fairbourn and James Therrian for layout and publishing consultation.

We have also been blessed with creative and smart research collaborators over the past thirty to forty years that formed the scientific base of the principles in the book: Co-investigators on the Family Health Projects, The Studies of Children's Activity and Nutrition, many studies on School Health, The CATCH (Coordinated Approach to Child Health) studies, and the NICHD Studies of the Early Child Care Research Network. There are too many to name, but special appreciation is acknowledged to Tom Baranowski, Jay Belsky, Robert Bradley, John Elder, Renate Houts, Russel Luepker, Thom McKenzie, Guy Parcel, Cheryl Perry, James Sallis, Elaine Stone, and Elizabeth Susman.

Finally, thanks to our own families and the many families we have been privileged to interact with over the years in both our home and professional lives.

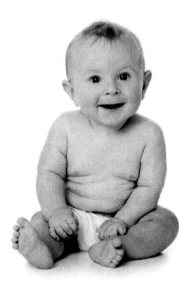

About the Authors

Philip R. Nader, M.D. is a nationally and internationally known Pediatrician expert in Child Development, Eating and Activity Behavior Researcher and grandfather. Michelle Zive, M.S., R.D., is a Nutritionist-writer and mother of two teenagers and a preschooler. Both understand this is not rocket science (Excess calories intake plus a sedentary lifestyle = weight gain). They have combined their expertise on community and family interventions and research on nutrition and physical activity, with sound principles of child development to bring parents easily understood tips and steps to take from the womb through adolescence in order to optimize the healthy development of their child.

Dr. Nader has a distinguished career of 30 plus years in community pediatric research and education. He has held tenured faculty positions at the University of Rochester, the University of Texas Medical Branch at Galveston, and the University of California at San Diego. He has led several multidisciplinary research teams investigating both epidemiological and randomized experimental trials dealing with childhood activity and nutrition. He continues his active research career as a Co-Investigator on the National Institute of Child Health Early Child Care Research Network with a focus on obesity and physical activity.

Dr. Nader served as Chair of the Data and Safety Monitoring Board for TODAY (Treatment and Prevention of Type Two Diabetes Among Youth) for the National Institutes of Health (NIH), and has served on other NIH clinical trials and ad hoc review groups. He has been active also in international community health efforts, having held a prestigious Fogarty Senior International fellowship in New Zealand and Australia. Locally in San Diego, he continues his community engagement through University and local efforts to prevent childhood obesity. He is a senior consultant with the San Diego County Obesity Initiative, and the Chula Vista Healthy Eating Active Community Initiative. He also serves on the External Advisory Board for the Consortium to Lower Obesity in Chicago Children.

Dr. Nader is known and respected among his peers, and has presented at national and international scientific meetings on childhood activity and nutrition in the United States, Australia, and New Zealand. He has published more than 150 peer- reviewed articles (see www.pubmed.gov). The article, "Identifying Risk for Obesity in Early Childhood", published in Pediatrics in September, 2006, received extensive media notice with well over 200 citations and stories in both print and electronic media. Subsequent to this publicity, major news networks now contact him to comment on other publications dealing with obesity. His special training as a behavioral pediatrician and as a parent of two and a grandparent of four helps to keep him grounded with practical ways for parents to fight the obesity epidemic.

Michelle Murphy Zive, M.S., R.D. has worked in community and nutrition research for the last twenty years in the Division of Community Pediatrics at the University of California, San Diego. Zive has been a contributing writer for the San Diego Family Magazine, where she's had numerous health articles published, including, with Dr. Nader a recent article, "Bye, Bye, Baby Fat," "Fighting Back: What San Diego is Doing to Combat Childhood Obesity," "You are What You Eat: Why Healthy Eating Habits are Vital to Adolescent and Teen Growth," "Exercise Your Influence Over Your Kid's PE," and "Prevent Childhood Obesity: What Parents can Do."

In addition, Zive has published in Salud Magazine, The San Diego Reader and a contributed to a book on "Opposing Viewpoints: Obesity."

She has been the director of a number of community and school nutrition and physical activity projects. She's published over fifty peer-reviewed articles on determinants of healthy eating and physical activity, as well as the impact of environment on health. In 1997/98, she was honored with the Excellence in Research Award from the California Dietetic Association.

Zive is the Principal Investigator of the Network for a Healthy California for San Diego and Imperial Counties, which is a collaborative program including over 100 public health organizations committed to helping people find ways to eat healthy and get enough physical activity.

As a mother of three, including two teen daughters and a preschool son, Zive's committed to sharing practical and easy tips and advice that she's learned throughout her career as a registered dietitian and researcher to inspire parents and others to help their children be the healthiest they can be.

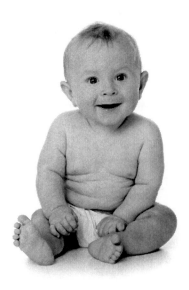